612.82   McKhann, Guy M.
MCK
          Keep your brain
          young.

$24.95

DATE			

KEEP YOUR BRAIN YOUNG

THE COMPLETE GUIDE TO PHYSICAL AND EMOTIONAL HEALTH AND LONGEVITY

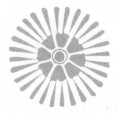

Guy McKhann, M.D.
Marilyn Albert, Ph.D.

John Wiley & Sons, Inc.

Published by John Wiley & Sons, Inc., New York
Published simultaneously in Canada

This publication is designed to provide accurate and authoritative information in regard to the subject matter covered. It is sold with the understanding that the publisher is not engaged in rendering professional services. If professional advice or other expert assistance is required, the services of a competent professional person should be sought.

Library of Congress Cataloging-in-Publication Data

McKhann, Guy M.
   Keep your brain young : the complete guide to physical and emotional
health and longevity / Guy McKhann, Marilyn Albert.
      p. cm.
Includes bibliographical references and index.
   ISBN 0-471-40792-5
   1. Brain—Aging. 2. Longevity. I. Albert, Marilyn. II. Title.
   QP356 .M385 2002
   612.8'2—dc21
                                                  2001007725

Printed in the United States of America

10 9 8 7 6 5 4 3 2 1

Dedication

To David and Hillie Mahoney—
a remarkable couple and good friends who were always there when we
needed them.

David—a retired businessman who, as chairman of The Charles A. Dana
Foundation, brought excitement and vision to the promotion of brain
research. We all miss him.

Hillie—a partner with David in all his endeavors. She continues to bring
her unique talents to continuing David's vision, both individually and as
a director of the Dana Foundation and as president of the Harvard-
Mahoney Neuroscience Institute.

Contents

Acknowledgments

This book has been a long time in coming. Its inception was related to the many years we've spent talking with patients, disease advocacy groups, students, and young doctors about the brain and its disorders. Many of these people have either discussed parts of this book with us or read specific chapters—we cannot list them all.

We have also gotten advice from colleagues of ours with expertise in specific areas. Again, we cannot list them all; we would like to particularly acknowledge Dr. Carol Johns, Dr. Robert Wityk, Dr. Steve Riech, Dr. Bill Falk, Dr. Ray DePaulo, Dr. Kay Jamison, and Dr. Guy McKhann II.

We also asked relatives and friends to read parts of this book as we considered them a subset of our potential audience. We would particularly like to acknowledge Harry and Pam Harrick, Carolyn and Arthur Kofler, Jeannette Albert, Emily McKhann, and Jeanette Glover.

We have been guided throughout this endeavor by the advice and assistance of colleagues at The Charles A. Dana Foundation. These include Francis Harper, Barbara Gill, Barbara Rich, and the current chairman, William Safire, and the current president, Ed Rover. We'd particularly like to acknowledge the assistance of people at The Dana Press, Jane Nevins and her associate, Elizabeth Lasley. We also got editorial assistance from William Patrick and editorial guidance from Tom Miller and Mark Steven Long of John Wiley & Sons. Finally, we wish to acknowledge the continuing help and guidance of Susan L. Soohoo, our administrative assistant.

PART ONE

THE BRAIN AND EVERYDAY CONCERNS

HEALTHY BUT REALISTIC IN THE SECOND HALF

We hear every day that we are part of an aging population. More of us than ever before are living longer than our parents and grandparents. Of course, we want these added years to be good ones. We want to stay active and productive. We want to spend time doing things that we enjoy, including some of things we had less time for in the frenzy of our younger years. And we'd like to pursue these activities in good health, and in bodily comfort, as much as we possibly can.

Some people seem to glide through the second half of life. We've all heard about such individuals—they tend to make the news—and many of us are lucky enough to know a few of them personally. Time lies lightly on these people, who are often called "successful agers," as they play their sports, keep themselves up to date on current events, and take active roles in their families and communities.

And then, apparently, there are the rest of us. While wondering how to age successfully ourselves, we begin to notice troublesome changes. To our consternation we can't walk quite as fast as we used to, or bend down as easily. We suddenly need a new eyeglass prescription. We no longer sleep through the night. Are these changes normal, and do they plague the successful agers as well? Are there things that we can do to help us age more easily and gracefully?

The answer is found in a place where many people might not think to look for it: the brain.

If there is one thing that determines how fully we live at an older age, it is how well our brains work. This may come as a surprise to many who do not realize how much the brain does. Most people tend to relegate the brain to cognitive or thinking arenas only. The fact is, the brain is involved in almost everything we do. Of course it is the control center of our thinking. But it also powers our feelings and moods, our movements, our senses, and certain bodily functions not generally associated with higher mental faculties. The brain is even responsible for what would seem to be the other end of thinking—sleep.

This book, *Keep Your Brain Young*, will help you understand how the brain serves us in all of these ways, and more. It will guide you through the changes that can be expected as you get older and your nervous system matures—as well as providing some good ways to cope with these changes. Perhaps most important, *Keep Your Brain Young* will emphasize ways to keep your brain functions performing as well as possible for as long as possible. As you'll see, there is a lot that you can do to keep your edge as you get older. Some of these things are quite simple; some require more thought and time. We spend a lot of time fixing, redoing, reshaping, revising our hair and hair lines, our skin, and our bodies. Surely it's also time to think more directly about our brain and what we can do for it!

We are two doctors absorbed by the human story of getting older. We don't just specialize in the brain; we devote our professional lives to an area that most lay people (and too many doctors) view with trepidation or even fear: the second half of life. Most people can't appreciate the beauty of living this second half with a sense of composure—and a sense of humor, when at all possible. We've seen so much we like and believe in about the brain in the second half of life—and plenty of things to be careful about as well. But the important thing is that you can be in harmony with getting older, and our mission in these pages is to help you do it.

We believe that knowledge and understanding is the key to taking any action effectively, and minding your brain is no exception. In our practices at Massachusetts General Hospital and Johns Hopkins University, we daily see older people who feel as if they've been set down in an alien landscape. They've always been accustomed to having their minds and bodies work a certain way; suddenly that's changing, and they don't know what to expect. Many of our patients are familiar with the term "successful aging;" they may have read books or attended workshops on the subject. But while these programs make valid points about things like lifestyle, attitude, and activity, they usually neglect other realities of growing older—the precise realities that we are questioned about most closely. Our patients are worried that their occasional memory lapses may be a sign of Alzheimer's disease. They wonder why they suddenly have to go to the bathroom three times a night. They're not sure whether everything they read about vitamins and nutritional supplements is true.

Our aim in writing *Keep Your Brain Young* is to fill this gap—to give you a single reliable, comprehensive guide to the all the normal changes and, sometimes, illnesses that may come in the later years to the organ that is the true center of your sense of self and quality of life, the brain. At the same time, we'll tell you how to minimize these changes and enhance your mental and physical functioning—without underestimating the very important role that lifestyle and attitude play. As the brain gets older, it goes through changes that occur in almost everyone. Your memory isn't as sharp. You don't see quite so well. Your sleep patterns change. And—though you might not have been worrying about your brain in this context—your sex life isn't what it used to be. These changes are part of normal aging, and to keep them from having too big an impact you can take steps that include physical exercise, overhauling your diet, being careful about alcohol intake, and finding better ways to handle stress—to name just a few.

Some people, of course, experience more than just the normal variations with age. They develop conditions that cut deeply into memory, motion, speech, and sexual function. In other words, these are people in whom some illness has been superimposed, like Parkinson's disease or Alzheimer's disease, on top of the common changes that occur with age. If you, or someone you are close to, has this extra trouble (and more people do as age increases into the eighth and ninth decades), what you can do about these problems, both on your own and with your doctor's help, is changing rapidly—thanks to the remarkable recent advances in brain science and those over the horizon. Things that were only dreamed about just a few years ago are now medical accomplishments.

When we first became brain scientists, friends and colleagues often asked us, "Why do you want to be involved with brain diseases? All you can do is describe them, you can't treat them." If that opinion was ever valid, it certainly isn't now. In the last few years there have been new medications and surgical treatments for many brain-related problems. More important, there are myriad new approaches in the pipelines of many pharmaceutical companies. Ideas that sounded like science fiction a few years ago are soon to be tried, or are being tried, in humans: vaccines for Alzheimer's disease, stem cells for Parkinson's disease, localized magnetic stimulation for depression, introduction of genes to treat brain cancer, and more. All those years and dollars spent in research on brain disorders are now starting to pay off. It really is a "brave new world" for those who care about the brain.

Keep Your Brain Young will share with you these newest advances: those that help define the problem and those that indicate the best treatment. This approach lies at the very heart of those goals common to all readers, patients, caregivers, other family members, doctors, and nurses: finding strategies that offset symptoms, wherever possible, and improving long-term outcomes.

Not all ideas come from conventional medicine, either. In our modern era of instant communication, most of us hear about many so-called alternative or complementary approaches: diets, food supplements, vitamins and minerals, and physical exercise. But how do we sort out all these various health claims? Anecdotes and advertisements are not enough. Listening to some of these claims, a person might sometimes try to exist on warm water and a few raw vegetables! But our decisions must be based on evidence—facts about safety, purity of compounds, and proof of benefit. We will do our best to explain and evaluate these approaches. Since, what is best for one person may not be best for another, we talk about how you can individualize prevention and treatment.

We will also emphasize the great importance of having a positive attitude. A positive attitude not only has beneficial effects on how well your brain works, but it also influences how you respond to diseases of other organs such as heart disease and cancer. One of the questions we like to ask an older person is "On a good day, when you are feeling well, how old do you consider yourself?" The answer is always illuminating! Many people in their late eighties and even nineties, see themselves as being somewhere in their late fifties or early sixties. This attitude is often part of a good self-image—it's probably what helps them maintain their maximum level of functioning.

Already a revolution is under way. Each succeeding generation is showing more interest in maximizing brain function and is realizing that they have the responsibility for staying as brain-healthy as possible. Because of new knowledge and advanced preventive measures, old age for future generations will be very different from the way it has been in the past. Start maximizing your future now, if you haven't already. It is never too late!

CHAPTER 1

MAINTAINING YOUR MEMORY

When Marilyn's mother, Carolyn, returned from vacation, she would always call her own mother, Rose, then in her 90s, and ask what had gone on in the world while she was away. Rose, who read the newspaper every day and watched the news on television every night, would bring Carolyn up to date on the details of recent world events. There was never any reason to check Rose's summary, because she always had things straight. As we write, Carolyn, now 87 herself, is currently reading the biography of a recent political figure, and as she retells some of the most interesting parts of the book, she expands the description on the basis of her own recollection of events.

We think that Carolyn has an exceptional memory, but she doesn't think so. She regularly complains that her memory isn't what it used to be, and says that her biggest problem is coming up with names. At times she astounds us with the details of names and places from the past. At other times, a name that everyone knows will elude her. For example, we were recently talking about New York City, the city in which she was born and lived for most of her life. We were reminiscing about the political scene in the 1930s, and were surprised to see her struggle to come up with the name of the mayor at that time, La Guardia. She knew that he read the comics on the radio every Sunday morning and that the airport was named after him, but she could not come up with the name. A few minutes later, we were talking about something else and she suddenly laughed and said, "La Guardia—I knew that." This common experience is often called a "senior moment."

These are not the memory complaints we see in our clinic, but we see them in our day-to-day lives all the time. Recently Marilyn was at a meeting with people who knew that she studied memory and aging. During the meeting, one of the men was having difficulty coming up with a name and looked nervously at Marilyn. She smiled and said,

"That's normal—it happens to everyone." Everyone laughed, and appeared to relax.

From experiences like these, and from speaking with numerous older people, both in our research and at large public meetings, we know that one of the things older people worry about the most is whether these "senior moments" are a sign of a more serious problem. Their concern is that this is the first sign of Alzheimer's disease. The publicity about this disorder emphasizes that the earliest symptom of illness is trouble with memory. However, normal changes take place in memory as we age, and these are not harbingers of disease.

MEMORY CHANGES WITH AGE

In middle age many people start to notice that their memory seems to be slipping a bit. This is particularly true when they are tired or under stress. Naturally, they get worried that more serious troubles lie ahead. It is comforting to know that even as late as age 90, about one-third of both men and women can take in new information and recall it later every bit as well as they did when they were younger. For many of the other two-thirds, memory continues to function quite well. But that does not mean that there are not changes. The large majority of healthy older people can expect some changes in memory function, not limiting, but troubling to the individual experiencing them. These changes include taking longer to learn new things and having trouble remembering names and strings of numbers.

Learning Slower But Well

It takes longer for the average older person to take in new information and retain it. Actually, if it is a small amount of information, such as a phone number, then an older person will do just as well, if he or she is really paying attention. In contrast, with larger amounts of information, such as a set of directions to a new location or the story line of a new joke, an older person will typically require more time and more repetitions to remember these details accurately. But all the evidence indicates that if an older person takes the time to learn something well, he or she will remember it as accurately as someone many decades younger. Thus, although older people think they are forgetting things more easily, in fact, what is happening is that they are not learning them as well in the first place.

Our friend Ellen is a good example of this. She decided to learn Tai Chi, the Chinese exercise ritual, at the same time that her grandson wanted to take lessons so they took them together. During the first few weeks, it became clear that her grandson was learning the formal motor movements at a much faster rate than his grandmother. At first she felt discouraged, but being a determined person she decided to persevere. As it happened, her grandson had to go back to school and was unable to continue taking lessons. Over the next few months, Ellen learned all of the Tai Chi movement routines that her grandson had learned so quickly. When the grandson returned from school, he was amazed at his grandmother's skill. As Ellen proudly explained, "It took me longer but once I learned them they stuck."

Remembering Names

The most common complaint of an older person with an otherwise good memory, like Marilyn's mother, is difficulty coming up with names. We all have some difficulty with this, and it does worsen, as we get older. For instance, you recall that such and such a fellow lives in a white house, drives a red car, and has a black dog, but no matter how hard you try you can't come up with his name. Some minutes later, while you are talking or thinking about something entirely different, the name suddenly comes to mind. As we mentioned above, this is normal.

Names, in fact, are the most difficult things to remember, because they are entirely arbitrary. Mt. Everest could have been called Mt. Supreme, which would have made a lot more sense, but it isn't. The name Jack is an arbitrary label and two people with the same name may have very little in common—think of Jack Kennedy and Jack the Ripper. That's why a series of associations is the best way to help you recall the name. Remembering names takes work, and some people are better at it than others. Many of us, when we first meet a person, focus on who this person is and what he does—the actual name is of secondary interest. Not so for others, who immediately make the association of the name, face, distinctive job, or relation to other people they know. All these associations are linked to that person's name, making it that much easier to recall.

Remembering Numbers

Although older people most often complain about difficulty with names, if we dig beneath the surface, we find out that they also have difficulty recalling sequences of numbers. Like names, number sequences are arbitrary: Why should one number sequence represent your phone number and another the phone number of a close friend? Moreover, even if you learn these sequences well and use them frequently, occasionally you will draw a blank on the phone number of a friend or even your own. This phenomenon, like failing to coming up with a name, is normal.

People with Exceptional Memories

If you ask people who had exceptional memories when they were young if their memory is as good as it used to be, they usually say no, and they will be very specific about what they can no longer remember as well. For example, the physician who used to be able to read an article in a medical journal and tell you not only the contents of the article but also where certain things were on the page will regret that he can no longer do that. Likewise, the retired stockbroker who once could keep track of the daily changes in the prices of hundreds of stocks no longer feels able to do it. But it is not clear whether the physician's and broker's perception of their memory is correct; it may be that it takes daily practice to accomplish such feats, and perhaps, if they tried, they could still do it successfully. Although there have been many studies of memory changes with age, we actually do not know if people who had exceptional memory abilities when they were young maintain them, because the tests used to evaluate memory are too easy to present an effective challenge for these people.

We know a retired lawyer, in her sixties, who said that in her youth she had had a photographic memory. She could read a page and remember exactly what was on it. During school, she didn't think she had to try to remember things, she just took them in by reading, and they stuck. A few years ago, after being retired for many years while raising a family, she decided to take a literature course at a university. The first night of studying, she had to read the same page 23 times to retain the information. Her photographic memory seemed to be gone. As she studied, trying to remember what she had read and wondering what had happened to her, the tears rolled down her face. However, two months later, after studying hard, paying attention as she read, her photographic memory was back. She is not sure it is as good as it was when she was younger, but she has clearly improved from the early days of taking that course.

DIFFERENT KINDS OF MEMORIES

These stories make it sound as if memory is all one thing, but it is not. The problems that can occur with memory depend a lot on what type of memory you are talking about. The biggest difference in types of memories is between old memories and new memories.

New Memories vs. Old Memories

If someone learning something new is exposed to it only once, whether or not the information sticks will depend upon many factors. These include whether the new information is important, whether it is associated with something already familiar, and whether or not the person is paying attention.

The part of the brain that is essential for learning and retaining new information is a small seahorse-shaped area called the hippocampal region (from the Greek *hippocampus* meaning "seahorse"). The hippocampus is involved when someone is actively learning something new. Once the information is well learned, however, it is actually stored in a different location, the part of the brain called the cerebral cortex. Thus, someone remembering things that happened many years ago is retrieving them from the cerebral cortex.

Certain diseases of memory make this distinction very clear. In the early stage of Alzheimer's disease, where the damage is focused on the hippocampus, the difficulty is in making new memories, but old memories are preserved. An Alzheimer's patient at this point can remember past events quite well, but may be totally unable to learn anything new. In contrast, the disease in its late stages damages many parts of the cerebral cortex, and memories for past events are disrupted.

Emotions also affect how well a person remembers things. Their impact is powerful in situations that are particularly pleasurable, dangerous, or upsetting, where vivid memories persist for years or sometimes even a lifetime. For example, those of us who are old enough can remember precisely what we were doing when we first heard that President Kennedy had been shot—where we were, who we were talking to, maybe even what we were wearing. The same phenomenon will occur in relation to the attack on the World Trade Center. Memories of events with particular emotional or historical importance are also likely to be well entrenched because you think about them many times, reinforcing their memory circuits in the cerebral cortex.

Memory for Skills and Memory for Facts

Memories for skills are stored differently in the brain than are memories for facts. Riding a bicycle, hitting a golf ball, or dancing, are skills that, once learned well, are with us even after long intervals. These skills can be preserved in people who have difficulty learning new facts. A patient of ours has a memory problem that makes it impossible for him to continue to practice law, but he can and does play golf quite well, three or four times a week. However, he cannot fill out his scorecard or keep score for others; someone else has to do that. The current thinking is that memory for skills such as the motor acts required to play golf or tennis are stored throughout the brain, in areas different from memory for specific details that keep changing such as the score or even the names of who is playing.

HOW YOUR BRAIN FORMS MEMORIES

Can you drive your brain to be better than it is genetically programmed to be? Little evidence supports the possibility. However, it is clear that you can attain optimal functioning and maintain it by stimulating usage. Each nerve cell communicates with thousands of others. But when you form new memories, you strengthen a particular series of connections, the way a heavily trodden pathway in the woods becomes more visible and easier to follow. Among nerve cells, two different things are happening. First, changes take place in the physical connections between nerve cells to make one pathway easier to use than others. These changes occur at the very end of the pathway, at the synapses, where nerve cells connect with one another. Second, some of the chemicals released at the synapses, the neurotransmitters, are specialized for memory. One of these neurotransmitters is acetylcholine. As we will discuss, many of the drugs being developed to attempt to modify memory involve increasing the effectiveness of this neurotransmitter.

Mentally and physically stimulating activities promote this constant "rewiring" of the brain, strengthening its pathways and stimulating the production of substances required for the growth and maintenance of nerve cells. In some instances, brain cells will make new connections. More commonly the balance between existing connections is altered, by strengthening some and weakening others.

Years ago scientists thought of the brain as being "hard-wired," meaning that during development, nerve cells would assume their proper positions and make myriad interconnections. Once in place and interconnected, it was thought that nerve cells did not change. This notion is clearly wrong. Research in the last few years has shown that new nerve cells may even develop in areas of the adult brain, including the hippocampus, the area that is important for making new memories. No one knows what regulates this replenishment of nerve cells, but recent evidence suggests that one factor may be physical and mental activity.

Genetics of Memory

Genetics also plays a role in how well memory functions. The behavior of animals is a good example. Certain breeds of dog, such as Labradors, are supposed to be gentle but perhaps a little dumb, meaning they do not learn new information easily. German Shepherds, on the other hand, generally learn quickly but are not particularly gentle. The same phenomenon is well known in laboratory animals. Some strains of mice can be taught to find food in a maze much more easily than others. Now that we know that genes can be either more or less active, it is possible to breed mice that are selectively smart or dumb. This line of research is one of the approaches that may eventually lead to drugs that will enhance memory for people.

But what about us humans? Everybody knows of families in which multiple members live into old age, preserving their intellectual abilities to a remarkable degree. Is this all related to lifestyle, or are genetic factors involved? Are different individuals genetically endowed to preserve mental functions and others not? Although we do not know the answer to that question, two possibilities seem likely. Some people may simply not have genetic vulnerabilities that lead to diseases like Alzheimer's disease. On the other hand, they may have other genes working that protect their brains from the decline in the abilities of nerve cells to function normally. Research to explore these alternatives is already under way in animals, such as mice, in which the genetic properties can be manipulated.

IMPROVE YOUR MEMORY

You can use specific memory training techniques to make your memory better on a daily basis. You can improve your ability to take in new information and retain it by concentrating and adding structure, putting the new information within frameworks you already know or already use. Another strategy is to associate the new information with existing knowledge that is meaningful to you.

Concentrate

Many older people underuse their ability to concentrate on the thing they are trying to remember. It isn't that they can't focus attention, but they don't seem to take into account that learning takes work. For example, if you want to learn how to use a new VCR or a computer, you have to concentrate. That means you may have to shut off the radio or avoid being interrupted in order to focus on the task at hand. Reinforcing information as you take it in is also helpful for retaining it. To learn a set of instructions to a new location, for instance, repeat the directions out loud. Develop the habit of actively paying attention. Just by concentrating on what you want to remember, your memory will improve dramatically.

Make Learning Conscious and Deliberate

Make a point of thinking to yourself that you want to remember something. Repeat what you want to remember to yourself. It doesn't take extra time to think to yourself, "I am parking my car next to the pole with the number 3 on it."

Don't Overload Your Circuits

Another change comes with getting older that can have an impact on memory. That is the ability to switch from one subject to another. For example, if you are on the telephone and someone comes into the room and tells you, "Call Marge," you may forget the message even though you heard it and understood it, because you were thinking about the telephone conversation. If two sets of information are in direct competition, older people tend to select one to remember and disregard the other. Younger people try to remember both and may remember less of either set, but they don't disregard one thing completely. For older people who are still working, this may be a particular problem, since our modern lifestyle is often quite hectic, with repeated interruptions and multiple things going on simultaneously. Making lists or notes can help. If, instead of trying to remember the message someone is giving while you are on the telephone, you make a written note, "Call Marge," to remind yourself, then the problem is solved.

Adopt Useful Memory Strategies

Use tried-and-true memory strategies. You can use very focused techniques, such as those taught in memory training courses. Putting the information you are trying to learn into chunks of five to seven items makes it easier to remember. Thus, if you can reduce fifteen names to three groups of five, it is easier for you to learn and remember them, just as it is easier to remember a long list of grocery items if you break the list into categories such as cleaning products, meats, and vegetables. It's no accident that telephone numbers are presented and written as chunks of numbers, and we remember them that way—(781) 252-8586 instead of 7812528586.

Another technique for improving your memory in this way has been attributed to ancient Chinese scholars; it involves imagining objects or names of people in specific rooms of a house. In this technique, you might put five names in the living room, five names in the kitchen, and five names in the bedroom. You then have to remember the relatively small number of people in each room. What you have actually done in using this technique is to take a large amount of information and break it down into small chunks, each of which you then associate with specific locations.

Make a Mental Picture

You may find it useful to make a mental picture of the thing you are trying to remember. If you want to be sure to remember where you parked your car, try to form a mental image of what end of the lot you are in, where you are in relation to the entrance to a store, which direction your car is facing, and signs or aisle numbers that are posted near the car. Strangely enough, it is more important to do this in a place where you park often than in a place you rarely go. When you come repeatedly to the same parking lot, with your mind on other things, you can easily forget where you parked. But because a new place is unfamiliar, you are much more likely to pay attention and make a special effort to focus on cues that help you remember.

Business or political leaders often use a similar technique when they are trying to concentrate on remembering which constituents were at a meeting. They will imagine them sitting around a table; later, this will help them remember who was at a meeting and what their names were. Making a mental picture of something may also help with everyday reminders. For example, if you want to remember to make a phone call when you get home, visualize a phone hanging in front of your door. When you see your door, it may remind you to make the call.

Use Pattern Recognition

If two chess players interrupt their game and leave the pieces on the board, a novice player can look at the board for 30 seconds to a minute and an hour later would be lucky to remember where four or five pieces were. An experienced chess player, however, can look at the board and give it a structure because of his knowledge of how the game is played, and be able to tell you where all the pieces were. However, if chess pieces are just randomly placed around the board, with no relationship to the rules of chess, a grand master will not remember any better than the novice where the pieces were. These chess pieces have been arranged in a way that is meaningless to his memory patterns based on the rules of chess structure. It is this ability to use structure that allows a master player to compete with 20 people at a time or to play chess blindfolded—or without a board. A similar phenomenon occurs with bridge players. Master bridge players can tell you about hands they played years ago. Their ability to use their memory is no better than anyone else's in other areas, but in analyzing bridge hands, they have developed a specific structure that allows them to perform these memory feats. In everyday life, we often use patterns to remember locations; for example, we may talk about the new store that is close to where the old one used to be. In doing this, we are using an old pattern of relationships to help us learn a new one.

Guy once asked a famous cellist whether, if when he tried to play a piece of music he had not played for years, he saw it, heard it, or just felt it in his fingers? He could not answer, and a year went by before Guy saw him again. The cellist shook his head in dismay when he told Guy that he had ruined a year of his life as he tried to find an answer to the question. He was unable to determine what conscious mechanisms he used to remember music. Probably it was a combination of all three—an example of the linkage of sight, sound, and tactile memories.

Make Associations

It's also helpful to make associations with the thing you are trying to remember. Marilyn's birthday is July 14, Bastille Day—French Independence Day; Guy's birthday is March 20—the last day of winter. At least one excuse for forgetting the other's birthday has been eliminated. Birthdays of grandchildren—they're another matter.

Some people find that thinking of words that rhyme with a name or attaching a word to a color or some important occasion helps them remember it. It is best to be sure that the associations are clear and resonant for you, even if for no one else.

Ways to Remember Names

For some people, remembering names is very important professionally, especially politicians or salespeople, and we can learn from their techniques. First of all, they pay close attention when they are hearing or seeing the name. Second, they try to repeat the name, usually out loud, thus reinforcing it in their mind. Third, politicians and business people often make an association right on the spot; they may say, "Oh yes, John, you live in Charlestown, right near the Bunker Hill Monument." So now this person becomes John from Bunker Hill. If you were part of a social or religious group, for example, you might use the same strategy when you meet a new acquaintance, such as the man who used to be an automobile dealer in Colorado. If you associate his name with his former residence and profession, you are reinforcing his identity three different ways. The reason this strategy helps is that memory is embedded within many different connections in the brain. The more associations, the more possible pathways are involved, and thus, the more likely you are to retrieve it later on. When you have trouble coming up with a person's name, you usually remember lots of facts about him or her. To remember the name better in the future, you need to imbed these facts as clues to it. Try repeating the name in your mind along with some memory-jogger about their profession or appearance—or even where the person is standing in the room.

Ways to Remember Numbers

Unfortunately, number sequences are becoming an increasing part of our daily lives, with repeated requirements for security codes for bank accounts, credit cards, and home security systems. One of the ways that people try to get around this is to use numbers that are meaningful, such as birthdays or anniversaries for the base of the number sequence. However, security companies recommend that you not use such numbers because they are easy for a third party to discover. An alternative is to use words that can be transformed into a number sequence, by substituting letters with numbers (for example, using f-a-c-e as the cue for 6135). We are amused by the computer-savvy people who suggest that we change our number codes frequently, so that others won't figure them out. Who's kidding whom? We have enough trouble with the ATM machine as it is.

How to Remember Facts

You can also use a phrase to help you remember facts. For example, "spring forward, fall back" helps most people remember which way the time changes in the spring and fall.

Write It Down

Make lists, use a calendar, or make notes. Why keep everything in your head? Writing notes and lists is a good technique for helping us adapt to the fact that it generally takes longer to learn new things as we get older. Sometimes just the act of writing something down helps you remember it better. For example, remembering directions to a new location can be difficult. It's embarrassing to keep asking the person to repeat them. Why not just say, "Speak slowly. I am writing this down"?

Organize Important Things

Put important items in the same place all the time so they will be easy to find. For example, always put your car keys on the table by the front door. This results in you having an association in your mind between the table and what you expect to be on the table. Thus when the issue of the car keys comes up, this association is immediately activated—a much better scenario than mentally retracing your steps.

Plan Ahead

In our experience, when successful older people have appointments, they tend to be early rather than late. This is because they are concerned about the various steps involved in getting to an unfamiliar location and make allowances for possible problems along the way. This ability to plan ahead is a good way for older people to adapt to the fact that they may move more slowly, may have trouble reading signs, and tend to worry that, if they make a mistake, it may take them longer to correct. Thus, by planning ahead, the successful older person avoids what could be a stressful circumstance.

DEVELOP A LIFESTYLE THAT CONTRIBUTES TO GOOD MEMORY

How you live your life on a daily basis makes a difference in how well your memory ability is maintained. What research has shown us, and what we hope to show you, is that there are simple steps one can take to stay mentally and physically young. For example, we helped conduct a large community study to examine what factors determine the maintenance of cognitive functions, particularly memory. As part of this study, funded by the MacArthur Foundation, our research group examined, with brief evaluations of mental and physical ability, 3,000 individuals and identified about 1,200 between the ages of 70 and 80 who were performing in the top third of the population in this age group. We kept track of these individuals for the next 10 years. Some people at the end of that time had preserved excellent mental functioning, while others had not. Three factors characterized those who maintained their mental abilities over time:

1. They were more mentally active.
2. They were more physically active.
3. They maintained a sense of effectiveness in the world around them, meaning that they continued to maintain a sense of control over their lives, felt that they were contributing to their family or to society, and generally felt good about themselves, too.

What is even better is that you don't have to do anything so very special to keep your mind in shape. Those who maintained their mental abilities kept their minds active through such stimulating activities as reading books, doing crossword puzzles, using a computer, and going to lectures or concerts. It is worth noting that the group better at maintaining their mental abilities was less likely to spend time in the passive mode of watching television.

Today, more people than ever are interested in programs related to lifelong learning and brain exercises. Someone has even coined a new word, "neurobics," to designate brain mental exercises. But it probably doesn't make any difference what program you use, so long as you get away from the TV set and interact with other people and exercise your brain in challenging ways.

Likewise, the physical activities the high-functioning 70- and 80-year-olds performed were everyday things—walking a mile or going up and down stairs. The important thing seemed to be that they did these activities regularly, not sporadically. They also had a positive attitude about life—feeling that they had an impact on their world and how they lived. For more on exercise, see the sidebar "What You Can Do about Memory: The Role of the Physical," on page 22.

We believe that people who maintain their sense of effectiveness are individuals who know how to adapt to life's challenges, rather than becoming overwhelmed by stressful situations. In addition, they maintain some degree of control in their daily lives, and are not overly dependent on others.

We can't prove this, but it may be that women not only live longer but possibly maintain their brain functions better than most men, in part because they shop. While shopping, they are physically active, wandering through stores carrying parcels. They are mentally active, comparing prices and making choices. And, after completing their shopping, they feel they have accomplished something.

Another important aspect of attitude and outlook is the ability to handle stress. Stress can both improve and interfere with the ability to learn and use new information. Low levels of stress make a person more alert and able to concentrate. Many successful people have found that a certain level of stress gets them cranked up to get a job done. These are the type of people who often leave the preparation of a presentation or a report to the last minute, and then devote all their energy to its completion. However, when stress levels become too high their functioning may get worse, particularly their memory and their ability to concentrate. In addition, research indicates that prolonged high levels of stress may even be harmful to the brain. Experimental animals that are exposed to high levels of continuing stress develop elevations in a hormone called cortisol, which is made by the adrenal gland. In these animals, high levels of cortisol have produced damage to brain regions important for memory. In people who have high levels of cortisol, similar areas of the brain can become shrunken. This suggests that stress may be directly responsible for these alterations in the parts of the brain important for memory.

We think that levels of cortisol are influenced by how you respond to stress. We all have stress in our lives; the trick is not let it overwhelm you. As we discuss in chapter 4, "Managing Stress," this means trying to develop strategies to limit and relieve the stress. That means not adding more stress unnecessarily, sharing some responsibilities with others, and seeking emotional support.

MEMORY DRUGS

Everyone would like to have a "smart pill" that would immediately make your memory better. No such pill exists right now, but researchers are studying a number of substances that may have effects on reducing memory loss associated with aging. In recent years the question of whether or not hormones, particularly estrogen, can either improve memory or prevent memory loss has received a great deal of attention. Hormones are substances made in one organ of the body and released into the blood, that then have effects on other organs in the body. Some hormones are made in the brain, others in organs such as the thyroid gland or ovaries. As people get older, the production of some hormones decreases. This is particularly striking in women at the time of menopause, when the production of estrogen markedly decreases.

Estrogen

Studies have suggested that estrogen reduces the likelihood of memory problems or of memory disorders, such as Alzheimer's disease. As we write at least two large studies are being carried out, comparing women on and off estrogen for a long period of time. The results of these studies will give a better idea about whether estrogen is clearly beneficial in terms of altering the memory loss of normal aging or delaying Alzheimer's disease. Of course, other reasons come into play for either taking or not taking estrogen. As literature about estrogen takes care to point out, the hormone has benefits in reducing osteoporosis, the thinning of bones that occurs as women get older. On the other hand, estrogen increases the chances of developing breast cancer in some women. Before rushing out and taking estrogen, you should take seriously some oft-repeated advice: discuss all these issues with your doctor.

On a positive note, because of the way estrogen attaches to different receptors in different organs, it may be possible for scientists to make a form of estrogen that affects only the brain. When that is done, this modified form of estrogen might protect the brain from aging without influencing risk for breast cancer.

Testosterone

The male hormone, testosterone, appears not to affect memory. The decline of testosterone in aging men is gradual, and highly variable. It is possible to determine whether testosterone levels are low by measuring blood levels. Ordinarily, older men do not take hormone replacement, but a few studies have compared men taking testosterone with those not taking it. The results of these few studies suggest that supplemental testosterone does not improve memory. That may be just as well, because testosterone can be associated with cancer of the prostate in some men.

Melatonin

Melatonin is a substance that we usually associate with sleep, but it also has other properties, including the regulation of other brain hormones. It is made in a small area of the brain called the pineal gland. As people get older the pineal gland shrinks, and less melatonin is made, meaning that older people become relatively melatonin deficient. Only a few studies have looked at the use of melatonin to help memory, but they suggest that this compound may help those who are having both sleeping and memory problems. Melatonin improves sleep and thereby reduces memory problems related to sleep loss. Whether or not it also has direct effects on memory functions is not clear.

MEMORY FOODS

One of the questions we are commonly asked is: "Is there any special food or diet that I can eat that will improve my memory?" Clearly, if such a diet existed, everyone who has trouble finding his car keys would want to be on it. We know of no such diet that will improve your memory. However, some dietary substances can help maintain your memory, and we discuss these in chapter 2, "Nutrition for the Brain: Food, Fuel, and Protection."

RESEARCH ON MEMORY AND AGE

As they get older, people care more about retaining their memory ability than about almost anything else. This has spurred a great deal of interest in memory research that is already leading to new insights. Working with experimental animals that can be genetically manipulated, scientists are uncovering basic mechanisms of memory. For example, in one study researchers have created "smart mice" by introducing a gene that increases the function of a receptor for a neurotransmitter involved in memory. This study is, undoubtedly, the forerunner of many others that will examine the basic mechanisms of memory that could lead to drugs that would enhance memory.

As we will discuss in other sections of the book, brain scientists are making an intense effort to find out not only how treat diseases of the brain, such as Alzheimer's disease or Parkinson's disease, but also how to prevent them. Similarly, everyone has an increasing interest in how to maintain a healthy brain, and in particular, good memory. Pharmaceutical companies have, up until now, been concentrating on drugs that modify one specific neurotransmitter (acetylcholine). They are beginning to branch out into other areas, considering other neurotransmitters as well as substances that nerve cells require for their normal maintenance and repair (so-called trophic factors). Most of these drugs are being evaluated to determine if they will prevent declining memory in dementing disorders, such as Alzheimer's disease. It is, however, inevitable that these compounds will also be tried to see if some of the "normal" changes in memory we described here can be modified.

WHAT YOU CAN DO ABOUT MEMORY: THE ROLE OF THE PHYSICAL

Scientists are beginning to trace the connections between mental and physical exercise and are learning how the two work together to help maintain mental ability. Several findings from animal research give us hints about what might be going on. More mentally and physically active animals show more elaborate connections between nerve cells and they have increased blood supply to their brain. Physical activity also increases at least one chemical in the brain that protects the brain and helps it grow; this chemical is called nerve growth factor. Some evidence even suggests that these changes are selective, helping some parts of the brain more than others. One brain region where physical and mental activity may make a big difference is the frontal lobes, the brain region vital to helping us focus on what is important and ignore things that are not, a vital aspect of learning and remembering new information.

A regular routine of moderate exercise provides structure, which is one of the pillars of good memory. If your exercise of choice takes you outdoors or into the company of others, it can be mentally stimulating as well, helping you work your navigational, organizational, and name-and-face remembering skills along with your heart and muscles.

Other physical factors play a role in mental acuity. Some daily habits can interfere with memory and other mental processes. These include excess alcohol, chronic lack of sleep, and many types of medications, particularly those used to promote sleep. These factors are often overlooked because they are not thought of as affecting general thinking ability. They are particularly important, because they are behaviors you can change, and their effects are reversible.

CHAPTER 2

NUTRITION FOR THE BRAIN: FOOD, FUEL, AND PROTECTION

Molly has always been very interested in nutrition. For years, she has paid close attention to good nutrition in general—fresh foods grown without pesticides, packaged foods without additives, and a healthful, well-rounded diet. Lately, she has become particularly interested in how nutrition might improve her memory. She does not want a pharmaceutical product for this purpose; she would prefer to use alternative medicines, such as herbal preparations. She has talked to us about vitamin E, gingko, and lesser-known preparations that claim to improve memory and has called us to check out several special diets and medications. Once upon a time, Molly's attention to foods and herbals would have been considered eccentric, but not anymore.

The whole question of nutrition and aging has become very interesting scientifically: What you eat does influence your brain's function; conversely, your brain helps to regulate when and how much you eat. Are there "brain foods" or dietary supplements that will make your brain function better or prevent cognitive decline? If you haven't been one to take an interest in these questions, we think you should "stay tuned"—for anyone in pursuit of successful aging, it's a busy new area of science and well worth watching.

GENERAL DIET AND MENTAL FUNCTION

If you are wishing you could organize your diet to pump up your perfectly normal brain to whiz-kid levels, the news may be disappointing. Very little evidence indicates that anything you eat will make a normal brain perform with superior intelligence or memory. Some evidence suggests that getting your blood sugar higher than normal will improve mental functioning for a short time. But, unless you plan to weigh 300 pounds or more, this isn't a very practical for the long haul.

A well-balanced diet provides the nutritional basis for what your brain needs. Beyond that, what evidence points to certain foods that are bad for you, or, on the other hand, foods that might be protective? Most of the attention paid to diet has focused on the types of fats and levels of cholesterol. You do want to watch out for too much saturated fat, such as animal fat, and too much cholesterol. Both are associated with diseases of the heart and blood vessels, the risk of stroke, and, some researchers believe, a relationship with Alzheimer's disease as well. In contrast, you can help guard yourself against heart disease by emphasizing unsaturated fats from such foods as fish (now often labeled as foods with omega-3 fatty acids). Consequently, since blood vessel disease plays a major role in both stroke and certain kinds of dementias, it makes sense to develop a habit of following a low-cholesterol, low animal-fat diet.

VITAMINS

Your brain also needs vitamins, but cannot make its own: most of the vitamins in your blood (and brain) come from your diet. And, as we all know from reading the sides of cereal boxes, you need certain minimum daily intake of vitamins for normal function of your brain and your body.

Vitamin Deficiencies

If you are eating a well-balanced diet, particularly if you add to that a general vitamin supplement, you will not become vitamin deficient, with one exception: some people cannot absorb vitamin B12, which plays an important role in the brain. In order for your body to use vitamin B12, whether you get it from food or take a vitamin supplement, you need to have a special substance produced by your stomach that promotes its absorption. For many people, as they get older their stomachs no longer produce this substance. Without it, whether you take vitamin B12 pills or food enriched with vitamin B12, the vitamin will pass right out of your system. If your stomach can't absorb vitamin B12, then you must take it by injection. Deficiency in this vitamin causes problems in both thinking and walking and prevents the normal formation of red blood cells, a condition known as pernicious anemia. Fortunately, B12 deficiency will show up in a simple blood test, and treatment is also easy: an injection of B12 once a month.

Apart from a vitamin B12 problem, vitamin deficiencies occur primarily when eating habits are abnormal. This is most common in heavy drinkers; they fill up on alcohol and don't maintain a normal diet. The calories in alcohol are called "empty" calories because they lack the proteins, vitamins, and other nutritional substances people need. The resulting vitamin deficiency, which is usually a thiamin deficiency, can be very sneaky. The symptoms—confusion, memory problems, and difficulties walking—may come on very gradually. And because family members and friends are often not aware of how much someone is drinking, they may not think of a vitamin deficiency as the explanation. If caught in time, this condition is readily treatable by eliminating alcohol and adding vitamins and proper diet.

Vitamins as Potential Treatments for the Brain

As your brain burns fuel, such as sugar and oxygen, some by-products accumulate, just as soot gradually accumulates in a furnace. The burning is called oxidation; the by-products are particles called free radicals, a form of oxygen altered so that it always wants to combine with substances in the membranes of nerve cells. This "sticking" to nerve cells not only damages how they function but eventually kills them. Some substances, particularly vitamin C and vitamin E, can mop up free radicals formed by oxidation. Thus, they are called antioxidants.

In recent years, advocates of nutritional approaches have encouraged the use of antioxidant vitamins in much larger doses than the minimum daily requirement for the prevention or treatment of brain disorders such as Alzheimer's disease or Parkinson's disease. In this, we agree.

Vitamin E

We see increasing reason to recommend vitamin E for daily use. That's because studies show that it delays the onset and may slow the progression of Alzheimer's disease; it may also lower the risk of other degenerative diseases such as Parkinson's disease. It is not clear whether vitamin E will actually prevent these memory problems or disorders or can reduce memory problems in normal people, but new studies currently going on may answer these questions. Despite that uncertainty, we recommend taking 1,000 units of vitamin E daily, because such a dose almost never has side effects and the evidence for its effectiveness is increasing. In addition, it doesn't tend to interact with other commonly used medications, such as blood thinners or aspirin.

Vitamin C

Although vitamin C is also an antioxidant, the case for it as a brain protector is not as strong as for vitamin E. A large study is evaluating the role of vitamin C in preserving brain function. We should know sometime in the next few years if it is of benefit.

Co-enzyme Q10

Co-enzyme Q10, sometimes called vitamin Q10, has a special role in maintaining healthy mitochondria, the small packets of enzymes that produce energy in all cells. Many physicians prescribe co-enzyme Q10 for prevention of heart disease. Its beneficial role may well extend to the brain: One of the conditions suspected of underlying Parkinson's disease is a deficiency in how mitochondria function. That suspicion is strong enough that studies are in progress to determine if co-enzyme Q10 can either prevent or slow the progression of Parkinson's disease.

HERBAL PREPARATIONS

Herbal preparations have received enormous attention as potential preventive strategies or treatments for age-related problems or changes in the brain. A visit to your local health food store or pharmacy will help you appreciate the large variety of herbal diet supplements available. Herbals have become a genuinely big business in the last few years. By some estimates, at least one-third of Americans have tried herbal medicines, for which they spend at least $3 billion per year.

The major difficulty with this burgeoning area is the scarcity of systematic studies to tell us which of these preparations really work. How do you know whether these compounds are what they claim? You should ask three basic questions about any health product you take: What is in it? Is it safe? Is there any evidence that it works? Let's look at these three important questions.

For conventional drugs, the Food and Drug Administration (the FDA), requires the manufacturers to have and disclose this information about any drug, old or new. For preparations classified as dietary supplements, no such protection exists. As long as the manufacturers do not claim to cure a specific disease, they can say whatever they want. For example, they can (and do) claim that ginkgo biloba helps memory, but they cannot say that it will cure Alzheimer's disease.

What Are the Contents of Herbal Preparations?

Unlike the manufacturers of regulated drugs and medications, the firms that make herbals are under no mandate to accurately list the contents, so with most dietary supplements you cannot trust the label in the same way you would trust the label on a conventional medicine or vitamin preparation.

In Guy's desk drawer is a bottle labeled "L-Tryptophan" to remind him how dangerous these unknown products can be. L-Tryptophan, a naturally occurring amino acid, was a preparation widely sold for sleep in the late 1980s. Unfortunately some batches of this product contained contaminants that caused a peculiar inflammation of the muscles that led to pain, stiffness, and immobility. This muscle disease would progress long after a person stopped taking L-Tryptophan, so hundreds of people were disabled by this compound before clinicians could figure out the cause.

Even preparations of a commonly used substance such as melatonin (popular for bringing on sleep) may vary from the label's list of contents. Not only may the compounds vary in their amounts of melatonin, but they also differ in additional ingredients. Another widely used product, DHEA, a hormone touted to slow aging, is also quite variable. A researcher obtained several samples of DHEA from a health food store and analyzed them. All had essentially the same label, but one contained no DHEA at all, while others contained 10 times more than the amount listed on the label.

Are Herbal Preparations Safe?

Conventional drugs have to be shown to be both safe and effective before they go on sale. This is done by testing the drugs first in animals and then in humans. Many conventional drugs have shown great promise in animal testing and preliminary testing in humans, but have flunked extended safety testing. These drugs either have not been brought to market or have been withdrawn after introduction. No such monitoring applies to alternative medications; these preparations stay on the market until some disaster occurs. Don't be swayed just because a product is called "natural"—L-Tryptophan certainly met that description. Many so-called natural products are extracted from vegetables, herbs, trees, and other sources, processed with chemicals, mixed with other substances, and turned into pills, oils, powders, or liquids of varying strengths, so there is nothing very "natural" about them.

Many herbal preparations can interact with conventional medicines. It is important to tell your physician or pharmacist what you are taking. Pharmacists have plenty of information in their computers about both conventional medications and herbal preparations and can look for possible interactions and precautions. The information in these computer databases should also be of enormous benefit as time goes on; it will provide more knowledge of which substances interact poorly with one another. Other information, available everywhere from the Internet to television commercials, may or may not be reliable. For tips on evaluating what you read, see "What You Can Do about Nutrition and the Brain: Don't Believe Everything You Read," page 37.

Are Herbal Preparations Effective?

With a conventional drug, effectiveness is determined by a clinical trial, usually involving at least hundreds of people. In clinical trials, one group receives the new drug and another group, called the control group, receives the standard treatment. If no standard treatment exists, the control patients receive a placebo, a sugar pill that looks (or an injection that seems) like the drug being tested. After everybody in the trial has been receiving the treatments for a length of time, the two groups are compared. If the new drug is better than the standard or nontreatment, the FDA approves the drug to be marketed for that specific use. No regulation requires manufacturers to prove the effectiveness of herbal preparations, thus they have no incentive to carry out similar clinical trials on their products. Competition might work as an incentive, except that advertising is usually a cheaper way to compete than clinical trials. That means, if we wanted to market a new herbal preparation that we claimed was good for the aging brain, let's call it "Brain Glo," we could do so as long as we didn't claim to cure any specific disease. It would be that simple and easy.

What Herbal Preparations Have Evidence for Effectiveness?

Only a few herbal compounds have been evaluated systematically for effectiveness in the same way as conventional medications—that is, comparing the herbal preparation against another substance. Depending on the clinical trial, this might be a comparison with a placebo or a conventional medication. Tested in this way and found to be effective are: ginkgo biloba for memory loss and dementia, fever-few for migraine, St. John's wort for mild depression, Asian ginseng for fatigue, and Valerian for insomnia. All these herbal preparations have multiple ingredients, so we are not able to say what is actually working and what the action is for any of them.

GINKGO BILOBA

The ginkgo tree (*Ginkgo biloba*) is one of the oldest species of tree on earth. It has been used for many years for medicinal purposes in Europe and has been a component of traditional Chinese medicines for centuries. It is probably the best studied of all the herbal medicines, and, as such, has several advantages over other herbal preparations. First of all, some of its components are known, and high-quality standardized extracts are available, particularly in German preparations. In the United States, ginkgo usually comes in crude preparations of uncertain strength.

Like many herbal preparations, ginkgo has attracted multiple claims, including that it will alleviate memory impairment, depression, and impotence. It is not clear whether ginkgo has beneficial effects for people with normal memory functions or with mild memory impairment. Ginkgo does, however, appear to have a modest beneficial effect in moderate-to-severe Alzheimer's disease—similar to drugs like Aricept (see chapter 14, "Treating Alzheimer's Disease and Other Dementias").

Ginkgo has remarkably few side effects, and is safe unless you are taking blood thinners, such as aspirin or warfarin. Ginkgo has some blood thinning properties and can increase the effects of these other medications. If you are taking ginkgo and expecting to have surgery, it is important to tell the surgeon because you could experience increased bleeding during surgery.

FEVERFEW

Feverfew is an herbal used to treat migraine and studies have associated it with fewer and less severe migraine attacks. The Canadian Health Production Agency (the Canadian counterpart of our FDA) has approved feverfew for the prevention of migraine on a short-term basis, but recommends its use for no longer than four months. As with ginkgo, you should not use feverfew if you take blood thinners.

ST. JOHN'S WORT

The German commission has approved St. John's wort ("wort" is an old English word for plant) for the treatment of anxiety and depression. In Germany, it is used about 20 times more commonly than Prozac, one of the most widely prescribed antidepressants in the United States. There has been only one study in the United States comparing St. John's wort with a placebo, and the results showed little benefit for those with more severe depression. We have prescribed St. John's wort with varying success for dozens of patients who could not take the usual antidepressants. The herb has many components, but hypericin seems to be the active antidepressant ingredient. If you want to use St. John's wort, it is important to use capsules that contain a known amount of hypericin and not a tea or other preparation that contains variable amounts of this ingredient. A study is comparing St. John's wort, the prescription drug Zoloft, and a placebo. The results of this study should be reported in 2003. St. John's wort may cause sensitivity to the sun, particularly in fair-skinned people, and this is a concern since skin cancer often develops in middle age and beyond. St. John's wort also may prolong the effects of anesthetic agents, so if you take it and have surgery scheduled, be sure to tell the surgeon about it. No studies have established whether it is safe to take St. John's wort with other antidepressants.

ASIAN GINSENG

The German regulators have approved Asian gingseng for treatment of fatigue and lassitude. Ginseng has also developed a popular reputation as an aphrodisiac, a claim backed by little scientific evidence. Ginseng is a striking example of the variations in herbal preparations: The amount of active ingredients varies, depending upon such things as the source of the plant, whether the roots or leaves were used, the age of the plant, the season it was harvested, and the method used to dry the plant. The magazine, *Consumer Reports,* compared 10 commercial preparations of ginseng. The amount of ginseng and of "gino-sides," considered to be the active ingredients, varied markedly from one preparation to another; one even had no active ingredients. Ginseng may have more side effects than other herbs, and you should avoid it if you have high blood pressure.

VALERIAN

The herbal valerian is a mild, nonaddictive sedative that improves both the quality of sleep and the time it takes to fall asleep. In Germany, valerian is approved for treating sleep disturbances. It is not known which of its many ingredients are responsible for its sedative effects. It is widely used in Europe and considered safe by the FDA of the United States. Valerian may prolong the effects of anesthetics, which means that, if you are taking it, it will take longer for you to wake up after surgery.

THE BRAIN NEEDS SUGAR

Bill came into the hospital for evaluation of pain in his feet. His physicians discovered the pain was due to diabetes, which was affecting the nerves to his feet. In diabetes, the body does not make enough insulin, the substance required to control the levels of sugar in the blood. The treatment is supplemental insulin.

While his physician was adjusting his insulin dosage, Bill suddenly had an episode in which he became sweaty, pale, anxious, and very confused. He did not know where he was, thought his physician was a prison guard, and became quite combative when she tried to reason with him. She tested Bill's blood sugar level, which was just one-quarter of normal. After she gave Bill some glucose in water to drink, he rapidly returned to normal. Had his blood sugar stayed that low much longer, he might have had convulsions or lost consciousness.

Like all organs, your brain requires food for energy and to build and maintain its cells. For the brain, the source of energy is glucose (sugar). The cells of other organs, such as muscle cells or liver cells, can use fats or proteins for energy, but not the brain. The brain has an absolute requirement for a steady supply of glucose.

The liver, pancreas, and kidney work together to maintain the right level of glucose in your blood. Your food and drink are broken down by your liver to form glucose. Your blood supplies glucose to your brain at a steady rate, which is essential for its functions. Too high a level of glucose in your blood, a state called hyperglycemia, will not have much effect on your brain. However, a level too low, known as hypoglycemia, causes problems in brain function.

Many people have the late morning or late afternoon blahs, when they simply run out of gas. They're suddenly tired, irritable, and can't concentrate. Often the problem can be solved simply by eating a snack that contains some sugar, such as fruit, at that low point in the day. Many people will have an improvement in memory and other mental functions for a short time after they take some sugar. This is entirely normal.

In contrast, we do see the rare individual who has significant hypoglycemia, whose levels of blood sugar can drop to as little as half of normal several hours after eating. Someone severely hypoglycemic may have headache, confusion, and systemic symptoms, such as sweating and a rapid heartbeat, when their blood sugar is low. Almost always, this kind of hypoglycemia has an underlying medical cause, such as the early stages of diabetes or other problems with the sugar balancing mechanisms, that need to be found and treated.

Prolonged fasting, such as for dieting or a religious ceremony, can have a similar effect. If you fast for 12 to 16 hours, a true hypoglycemia can develop, but it's transient and relieved by eating.

Hypoglycemia may even happen if you skip breakfast, putting an interval of 16 to 18 hours between dinner and lunch the following day. In these circumstances, the blood sugar level gradually drifts down, until the symptoms start to appear. Again, the treatment is to get the blood sugar up by eating. Studies comparing how well a person learns new information after skipping breakfast with how well the person learns after having eaten breakfast show that simply eating breakfast improves mental performance.

Most people with diabetes have learned to recognize symptoms of hypoglycemia and carry around some packets of sugar to take at the first sign of distress. Older people with both diabetes and cognitive impairment, however, may not be able to let others know their predicament or get to a supply of sugar. If you are taking care of someone with these problems, be aware of this potential for trouble. It is very easy to check the blood sugar with a pinprick and testing papers, if you can, but, when in doubt, it won't do any harm to give the person a little sugar in orange juice.

THE BRAIN NEEDS PROTEIN

Your brain needs glucose for energy. But to build cells, to produce chemicals necessary for nerves to communicate, and to repair damage, you need building blocks—proteins. The proteins you eat do not go directly into the brain because the brain is protected by a filter, called the "blood-brain barrier." Even though the level of some substance might be quite high in your blood, this filter keeps it from getting into your brain. Otherwise rapid fluctuations and surges of substances that might be helpful at low levels, but harmful at higher levels, would pummel your brain. The blood-brain barrier excludes from the brain many substances, including protein from the foods that you eat and medications, such as antibiotics. In contrast, other substances, such as glucose, pass freely into the brain. The more glucose in your blood, the more in your brain. Other substances do get into the brain but at slow, controlled rates.

Since proteins cannot pass directly into the brain, your brain makes it own, using the substances that do cross the blood-brain barrier, namely amino acids. Amino acids are the basic structural units of proteins, which combine together like beads on a string. When you eat protein, say, in soybeans or steak, your intestinal tract and liver digest it, breaking the protein's long strings of amino acids into individual amino acids, which circulate in your blood. Like glucose, these lone amino acids can enter the brain, which then assembles them to make the specific proteins it needs. At this level it does not make any difference to your brain if the source of protein is beef or soybeans.

APPETITE AND THE BRAIN

With such a smart brain, you want to watch your weight as you age, and not just to look good: Being overweight increases your risk for diabetes, heart disease, stroke, and some sleep disorders. If you're dieting, you're right in step with many others in the developed world; people are spending enormous amounts of time and energy trying to lose weight by eating less, eating differently, and taking special diet preparations. And, of course, we all are on an eternal search for a magic preparation that could help us lose weight and maintain that weight loss. Holding the line after losing weight is a particular problem because, of those who achieve their optimal weight after dieting, more than 75 percent regain the weight within two years.

The weight-loss yo-yo can be awfully tough. The role of the brain and genetic factors is greatly underappreciated in how body weight is regulated. Your brain receives two types of signals that influence your appetite. One tells you to stop eating during a meal; the other regulates how much you eat every day. The first is called a satiety signal and goes from your stomach and intestines to your brain. It signals the brain that you are full, and it is time to stop eating. The satiety signal takes time to develop; that is why you should eat more slowly, to give this signal time to kick in. If you eat quickly, you may well consume many more calories than you need before your brain can stop you.

The other signal is more leisurely and is generated from the cells in your body containing fat, your adipose tissue. These fat cells release a substance known as leptin into your blood, which tells your brain to decrease your appetite. The fat cells act like a thermostat in your home. When the temperature gets too high, the thermostat shuts off the heating system. Likewise, when your fat cells are full, they release leptin to signal the brain that you do not need to eat any more. However, when the temperature in your home drops, the heating system turns back on. Similarly, when you have less fat in your fat cells, as when you diet, your fat cells release less leptin, which your brain takes to mean that you need more food.

When leptin was discovered less than a decade ago, it aroused much excitement, not least because it pointed to a new mechanism for appetite control. Scenarios danced in scientists', magazine writers', and drug makers' heads: Maybe leptin would be the magic answer to diet control, and injections of leptin would decrease appetite and weight. It was not to be. Studies recruited overweight people to receive injections with either leptin or a placebo for two years. Disappointed researchers recorded only a small amount of weight loss and only in some of the people receiving leptin. The explanation may be that those who do not respond to leptin have genetic differences in how their nerve cells react to it. Once investigators thought about it, it didn't seem so surprising. After all, even certain strains of mice are very overweight because leptin has no effect on their brains.

Hope remains, however, that leptin can play a role in helping some people keep off the pounds they lose. Fat cells make less leptin after weight loss, and the leptin drop-off brings appetite surging back.

The hope is that after people with normal responses to leptin have lost weight, they could take leptin to keep their appetite from bouncing back. Studies are investigating this theory.

RESEARCH IN NUTRITION AND THE BRAIN

People of all ages like the idea of using nutritional substances to prevent normal aging changes that occur in the brain or to treat disorders of the brain. We all would benefit if standards for herbal preparations were higher. The rate at which Americans are trying them has attracted regulators' attention to the occasional hazards that are now showing up. We applaud this needed oversight. It might encourage manufacturers to do the necessary studies to establish that their plant products are both safe and effective. Many currently used medicines, such as drugs for the heart, antibiotics, and anticancer drugs, come from plants, and undoubtedly many more plant-derived products exist. The challenge is to find and properly evaluate these potentially effective substances.

Those of us in our middle years are especially interested in preventing changes in the brain with age that we used to (grudgingly) consider normal. Most of the new emphasis on preventing these changes focuses on substances such as vitamin E, which has antioxidant properties. But new antioxidants are "in the pipeline." Using experimental animals, pharmaceutical companies are developing antioxidants that can prevent the formation of free radicals or remove them. These new substances will soon be tested in people.

Another promising area of research is the development of nutritional products that will preserve the energy-producing mechanisms in the brain, the small packets of enzymes called mitochondria. These enzymes gradually change with age; their ability to produce energy in the brain diminishes. Specific diseases, such as Alzheimer's disease and Parkinson's disease, may also involve such changes in mitochondria. Substances under study (besides co-enzyme Q10 mentioned earlier) may help preserve normal function in the aging brain.

Scientists are just starting to understand the brain mechanisms that influence appetite and body weight. For example, exactly how leptin's signal decreases appetite is still unknown. When researchers find out more about it, trials of leptin-like compounds to control body weight, as well as attempts to modify the brain circuits involved in appetite control, will begin.

WHAT YOU CAN DO ABOUT NUTRITION AND THE BRAIN: DON'T BELIEVE EVERYTHING YOU READ

Hearing about herbals is easy, but finding reliable information about them is hard. One problem is that many magazine articles, books, TV advertisements, and now web sites are not as interested in informing you as trying to sell you something— a technique, a drug, or a combination of approaches. With no objective standards and few rules to go by, it is increasingly difficult to sort through all the claims.

Another problem is that some advertisements refer to, or show, an expert praising the benefits of the product. All too often, what is left unsaid is that this expert has a financial interest in the product. We feel that it should be mandatory to disclose that kind of vested interest.

But perhaps the biggest problem is finding out for yourself what claims are based on facts. A major source of health information today is health-related web sites. These sites are like a two-edged sword. A wealth of information is immediately available to you, much of it valuable. The problem is that anybody can say anything they want on a web site; they don't have to know what they are talking about. How can you tell what is valid? We recommend that you rely on sites associated with government agencies, major medical centers, universities, and respected health organizations, such as the American Heart Association. In the field of nutrition, Tufts University maintains one of the best sites (www.navigator.Tufts.edu). It gives you not only advice from Tufts's own experts but also their opinions of the accuracy of information at other sites.

The German government, unlike the United States government, has taken steps to monitor the safety and effectiveness of herbal preparations. Germany has formed a commission that periodically publishes evaluations and specific recommendations about herbal preparations used in Europe, such as ginkgo and ginseng. This publication is called the *Commission E Report*. Recently, several other organizations have published English-language reports based on the German report. The most comprehensive of these is the American Pharmaceutical Association *Practical Guide to Natural Medicines,* published in December 1999. Both the German and American publications recommend the products that have known amounts of ingredients and have been evaluated for safety and efficacy. They also tell you about side effects and possible interactions with other drugs.

CHAPTER 3

SLEEP AND THE BRAIN

DIFFERENT KINDS OF SLEEP

Until quite recently, sleep was considered simply a function to rest the mind and body from the day's efforts. We now know that sleep is a very active process. People are not unconscious during sleep; they remain responsive, particularly in their dreams.

Researchers had long noted that the eyes moved during sleep, but had missed the observation that eye movements came in bursts. Following these bursts of movement, the eyes were still again. When awakened during the rapid eye movement phases of sleep (called REM sleep), people reported that they had been dreaming. It has subsequently been shown that 80 percent of dreaming occurs during REM sleep. Sleep is now divided into two categories: REM sleep and non-REM sleep.

During REM sleep the brain performs in some surprising and contradictory ways. Nerve cells that are involved in the movements of eyes and facial muscles are turned on, thus permitting rapid movement of the eyes and twitches in other parts of the body. At the same time, nerve cells in the spinal cord are turned off, and thus the body as a whole will move very little during REM sleep. This turning off of nerve cells in the spinal cord has a protective purpose. People dreaming about running or swimming don't make the corresponding body movements. If they did, they might not only injure themselves but find it hard to convince a partner to share the same bed. During REM sleep, the heart rate goes up and the rate of respiration may increase. It has been suggested (but there is no way to prove it) that people who die during their sleep from heart attacks may do so during REM phases of sleep.

You have several periods of REM sleep during the night. When you first go to sleep, you do not go immediately into REM sleep. For 60 to 90 minutes you go through phases of lighter to deeper non-REM sleep and then cycle back to lighter non-REM sleep. At this point you make the transition into the first REM phase of the night. Each phase of REM sleep lasts from 5 to 30 minutes, and REM intervals recur 3 to 5 times each night. The pattern is irregular but usually the REM phases that occur in the later sleeping period last longer. It appears that people must spend a certain amount of time in REM sleep each night. In sleep research, if people are deliberately awakened during consecutive REM phases, they become "REM sleep deprived," and it becomes increasingly difficult to awaken them. When they are allowed to compensate, they spend much more time in REM sleep than they would normally. Some people deprived of REM sleep become more irritable and can exhibit pathological personality traits, including hallucinations.

Sleep Changes with Age

As people get older, a decrease begins in both the total time sleeping and the amount of time spent in the stage of sleep associated with dreaming (when REM occurs). A newborn sleeps 16 hours per day; during about one-half of this time, rapid eye movements are occurring. In contrast, the baby's 30-year-old mother sleeps 6½ hours per day (if she's lucky), and only one quarter of this time, or 2 hours, is occupied by the deepest stage of sleep. Starting in middle age (between 45 and 60) not only does the amount of sleep per night start to decrease but also the character of sleep changes. People these ages spend less time in the stage of sleep associated with dreaming and more time in the lighter stages. During the lighter stages of sleep, they are awakened more easily and spend time in bed in a twilight zone, feeling neither quite awake nor quite asleep.

As we mentioned in chapter 1, "Maintaining Your Memory," lack of sleep can interfere with memory. Several studies have shown that if you are sleep-deprived you will have more trouble than usual taking in new information and retrieving information you learned previously. There is no evidence that taking something to wake you up if you are sleep-deprived, such as amphetamines, will improve your performance.

Dreaming

One of our friends, in his 80s, recently had a cardiac pacemaker installed. At dinner at his house not long afterward, he commented about how much better he was sleeping, particularly about the marvelous dreams he was having. At that point in the conversation, his wife, who was of similar age, broke in and firmly said, "Dear, you are not going to tell them about those dreams." So we never did learn the content of those marvelous dreams.

Most of our dreaming occurs during the period of time when we have rapid eye movements, the REM phase of sleep. Researchers have found that the first phase of REM sleep contains relatively quiet dreams, whereas the phases of REM sleep closer to morning contain dreams that are longer and more intense. These are the dreams you are most likely to remember upon awakening.

People have been fascinated by the content of dreams since ancient times. Freud based his theory of the interpretation of dreams on the assumption that the ego relaxes its vigilance during sleep and the id, or instinct, allows forbidden wishes or drives to escape. In Freud's era it was believed that people had only a few dreams each night. One wonders what Freud's interpretation would be now, if he knew how much time people actually spend dreaming. A few studies have attempted to compare the content of dreams in the elderly with those of younger people. The elderly are less likely to have dreams that reflect day-to-day anxieties, like domestic or child problems, but are more likely to have issues of death in their dreams. In other words, not surprisingly, dreams reflect the life issues at various ages.

Nightmares are also familiar to all of us. They occur at all ages. They can occur during any phase of sleep, but the really violent nightmares, in which one awakens in a cold sweat, quite terrified, generally occur during the REM phase of sleep, as part of dreaming. In rare situations, older people may not have the normal inhibition of motor movements during a dream and may make violent movements, perhaps even getting out of bed and trying to run or thrash about. This change in sleeping behavior can be a danger not only to the sleeper, but also to a sleeping partner. A drug, such as Clonazepam, may be helpful in quieting these excess movements during dreaming.

What are the purposes of dreaming and sleeping? No one is certain, but theories abound. A popular speculation, backed by some studies, is that sleep is related to how the brain processes memories. This theory suggests that during sleep, the brain reorganizes and consolidates the information gained during the waking period. In addition, the brain might be strengthening new memories by reactivating the circuits that were involved in their original acquisition and processing. An alternative hypothesis is that that during sleep the brain erases the unimportant information accumulated during the day. Perhaps we dream and sleep in order to forget.

How Much Sleep Do You Need?

For most people between young adulthood and midlife, the total amount of sleep needed is seven to eight hours. However, people vary a lot in sleeping patterns. Some are "night owls," doing their best work late at night and in the wee hours of the morning. Others are "morning larks," up at dawn and having accomplished half a day's work before breakfast. Then there are those rare people who just seem to be able to get by on less sleep, maybe three to four hours a night. Some evidence suggests that "short sleepers" are more efficient in their sleeping behavior. They go into deep sleep (the rapid eye movement phase) faster and spend more time in this deep phase of sleep than do "long sleepers."

As people get older they are more likely to shift the time when they sleep, some going to bed and to sleep earlier and waking up earlier. Others are the opposite, staying up late into the night and sleeping much of the day. When people are in their 80s, these changes are even more pronounced. Their total time asleep per day may be only six or seven hours, including time spent in daytime naps. Even though a person may take several naps a day, the total time sleeping in naps is rarely over an hour. The idea that older individuals should sleep soundly for 8 to 10 hours is clearly wrong.

As a rule of thumb, 1 hour of sleep is required for 2 hours of being awake. As we get older, that ratio becomes closer to 45 minutes of sleep for each 2 hours awake. In other words, throughout the day you gradually accumulate a "sleep debt." By the end of a 16-hour day, a younger person owes the "sleep bank" 8 hours. In contrast, an older person has a sleep debt of only about 6 hours.

If you have been up for a long time and need to stay awake, you can use all kinds of tricks: going for a walk, taking a cool shower, or drinking caffeine in various forms. All of these may keep you awake, but they do not pay off your sleep debt. Many people, just dealing with the demands of everyday life, do not get enough sleep. By the end of a week, they may have accumulated a sleep debt of 8 to 10 hours. "Sleeping in" for an extra hour on Sunday morning will not pay off that debt. What will help you avoid a chronic sleep debt is to prevent over-scheduling your evenings, to allot time for sleeping, just as you do for exercise, work, and family.

We also have internal biological clocks, the internal pacemakers that govern the cyclical behavior of a number of the processes that give us daily cycles of higher and lower tendencies to sleep. The biological clock is the reason that we often feel tired at about three o'clock in the afternoon. The biological clock also leads us to have a strong drive to be awake at both 9 A.M. and 9 P.M. That is why it is often difficult to go to sleep early unless we are very tired or make it a habit.

Many people, without realizing it, are taking advantage of their biological clock when they have an afternoon nap. A brief nap can be very refreshing and improve functioning in the late afternoon and early evening.

TROUBLE SLEEPING AT NIGHT

People complain about many different problems with sleep, but the one that leads the list, and for which most people want a medication, is difficulty getting to sleep, and staying asleep, at night.

Difficulty Getting to Sleep

The most common cause of difficulty getting to sleep is the inability to shut off the anxieties and worries of the previous day. Sometimes it is a holdover from unpleasant events like an argument with a boss or family member; other times it is a pleasant event, and one is too "pumped up" to doze off. One of the authors is a football fan. Monday night football has been his downfall; after an exciting game, sleep is often hard to come by.

Some people have developed a habit of reviewing tomorrow's schedule just before they go to bed. They then toss and turn while they prepare for tomorrow's problems. The newest variation on this theme is taking one last look at e-mail messages on the computer, which is not necessarily a good way to put one's mind at rest. One way to get rid of these sleep-chasing proclivities is to make rules that will let you deliberately prepare for sleep, starting about 9 P.M. After that, no telephone calls, no more business, no late-night news, no planning for tomorrow's battles. For some, the mere thought of *trying* to go to sleep provokes anxiety. Going to bed and just lying there is not a good thing to do. It is better to wait until you feel sleepy.

Another common reason for difficulty getting to sleep is being in a new, unfamiliar environment. The noisy hotel room at a convention in a busy city or the guest room in a family member's home has all kinds of sounds and sensations that are unusual. This kind of tempo-rary problem getting to sleep is one situation where the brief use of sleeping medications, either over-the-counter or prescription, can be helpful.

Of course, caffeine can also be a problem. Either taken in coffee, *chocolate* tea, or sodas, caffeine is everywhere. The effect lasts longer than you think. It may be necessary to reduce or completely eliminate the use of caffeine, or at least stop it after noon, if you are having trouble sleeping.

Difficulty Staying Asleep

Difficulty staying asleep is a major problem in the elderly, and it gets worse as people get older. With sleep getting lighter and less time spent in the deeper phases of sleep, outside noises and distractions that would not disturb a younger person awaken someone older. In addi-tion, many more medical problems in the elderly can interfere with sleep. The pain associated with arthritis, back and neck discomfort, leg pain from diabetes, and leg cramps can awaken a person nightly, often requiring that a person get up, walk around, or even take some pain medicines. Those with asthma or poor heart function often awaken short of breath. Moreover, many medications can interfere with sleep, such as some high blood pressure medications, steroids, and antide-pressants. If you are suddenly having trouble staying asleep, a recent change in medication is one of the first places to look as a cause.

As people get older, it is almost assumed that they will not get through the night without going to the bathroom at least once or twice. This is particularly true when a person is taking heart medicines to remove excess water, so-called diuretics. If this "call of nature" is inevitable, the trick is to not let it be a pause that allows the day's anx-ieties to take hold and interfere with sleep for the next few hours.

Early Morning Awakening

A pattern of sleeping quite well until the early hours of the morning, and then awakening and not being able to go back to sleep, is the sleep disturbance we see most in depression. As we discuss in chapter 5, "Unmasking Depression," depression often goes unrecognized. This pattern of sleep disturbance should be a tip-off to the possible pres-ence of depression.

SLEEPINESS DURING THE DAYTIME

Many things can cause sleepiness during the daytime, including medications, jet lag, sleep deprivation from poor nightly sleep, or the need to be awake during the night.

Medications

The most widely used medications that produce daytime sleepiness as a side effect are antihistamines for allergies. Medicines used for depression, anxiety, and epilepsy can also cause sleepiness. If you are having trouble staying awake during the day, it is important to review the medications that you are taking to see if any of them may be the cause. The reason that many medications require a prescription for their use is because of sleepiness as a side effect.

Sleep Deprivation

As we mentioned earlier, if you don't allot enough time for sleep, you become sleep-deprived. Besides being sleepy during the daytime, sleep-deprived people often have problems with their thinking. They are slower to learn new things, may have problems with memory, and their ability to make judgments may be faulty, enough so that they may think they are really starting to "lose it," when the problem is really not enough sleep.

Elderly people do not recover from sleep deprivation as quickly as younger people. In experimental situations where people are kept awake kept awake for 24 hours, those in their 70s take at least a day longer to recover from their subsequent daytime sleepiness than younger people. Gender may also make a difference in the time it takes to recover from sleep deprivation; women seem to be able to recover faster than men.

JET LAG

The effects of jet lag are not just because you've deprived yourself of sleep with an overnight flight, but because you have confused your biological clock, which is still on home time. When you land in Paris on a flight from New York, you face a six-hour time change. Nine A.M. in Paris is 3 A.M. in New York, precisely the time when your New York-based biological clock is giving you the strongest signals to be asleep.

One spring, Guy, whose biological clock is set for Baltimore, had to make a business trip to Japan lasting four days. Since Japan is 12 hours ahead of Baltimore, trying to get his sleeping schedule adjusted was absolute murder. He found that he would awaken at about 4:00 A.M. and just could not get back to sleep. One of those mornings he turned on the television set in his room and, lo and behold, the Baltimore Orioles were playing the Detroit Tigers. He began to watch the game, thinking, "No one is going to believe this. Here I am sitting in Japan at four o'clock in the morning in my underwear, clutching a beer, watching the Orioles. I might as well be in the bleachers back in Baltimore!" At breakfast with the other two men on the trip a few hours later, there was a discussion of how they had spent the night. It turned out both had the same problem and had discovered the same baseball game on TV!

When you return home from a trip, disturbance in the sleep cycle continues, because your biological clock is somewhere in between. If your trip lasts for a few weeks, keep in mind most people require one day to recover from each hour of time change. People in their 60s and older who go on a vacation trip with these kinds of time changes should build this prolonged recovery time into their schedule on returning home.

Arousals from Sleep

Another reason for daytime sleepiness is having numerous brief arousals during the night, so-called "micro arousals". Despite being awakened very briefly many times during the night, usually the sleeper is totally unaware that sleep is being interrupted.

ABNORMAL LEG MOVEMENTS

Abnormal leg movements are a common but often unrecognized cause of micro arousals. They come in two forms, either or both of which may affect the same person.

In the first, called restless leg syndrome, a person has an uncomfortable sensation in the legs, usually from the knees down. The sensation is often described as burning, tingling, or the crawling of imaginary insects inside the legs. A distinctive feature is that the sensations get worse when the person tries to relax or lie down.

People with restless leg syndrome may have trouble falling asleep and staying asleep. But the sensation makes itself known at other times, too, particularly when sitting in confined spaces like airplane seats or desk chairs. The person has an overwhelming urge to get up and walk around, which sometimes can be a problem.

The syndrome can begin at any age but worsens as a person gets older. Some afflicted people have an underlying medical condition, such as diabetes. In most people, however, no cause can be found. In some rare families the problem crops up in successive generations, a pattern that indicates a dominantly inherited gene. As yet, scientists have not found such a gene.

Closely related to restless legs, and often occurring in the same person, are repetitive jerks of the legs while on the brink of falling asleep or in the early stages of sleep. These movements can disturb the sleeper, leading to poor sleep at night and excessive sleep during the day. In addition, a sleeping partner gets tired of being kicked.

Caffeine, alcohol, or smoking may aggravate both restless leg syndrome and nocturnal leg movements. The treatments, at least for some, are the medications used to treat Parkinson's disease (drugs that increase the action of dopamine, a neurotransmitter important in regulating movement).

LEG CRAMPS AND LEG PAIN

Leg cramps and other forms of leg pain are increasingly common as people get older. A person may be awakened from sleep by sudden pain and have to get up and walk around to relieve it. There are a variety of underlying causes. Some have abnormalities of nerves from diabetes, others have pressure on nerves from changes in the bones of the spine. In many people there is no obvious cause. Quinine, taken at night before going to bed, may help. Others find that calcium tablets, also taken at night, will prevent the cramps.

SLEEP APNEA

Someone suffering from sleep apnea will have noisy snoring and breathing that will slow down and may actually stop. The sleeper makes grunts and gasps for breath as if he is choking. If he is hooked up to heart and blood pressure monitors, the readouts can be quite frightening. The heart slows, and may even stop for a few seconds. After breathing starts again, the heart may race, and the blood pressure may shoot far above normal. These disturbances repeatedly arouse the sleeper for a brief period, and then the cycle starts all over again, without the sleeper being aware that any of this is happening. Some people may go through as many as 300 of these cycles each night.

What is happening is that for reasons that are not entirely clear, while attempting to breathe, the sleeper's upper airway, the back of the throat, becomes closed. The suction created by the diaphragm causes the upper breathing passages to collapse, and air cannot get through.

Sleep apnea is most common in overweight men over 65, but can occur in anyone. One of the easiest ways to detect this disorder is to put a tape recorder on the person's pillow and then listen for the distinctive pattern of loud snoring and alterations of breathing.

A friend of ours was so tired during the daytime and so worried about his memory that he came to us to be reassured that he was not developing Alzheimer's disease. When we quizzed him, we learned that he was constantly nodding off during the day, to the point that his wife refused to let him drive. We arranged to have his sleep monitored and discovered that he was awakening at least 200 times a night with episodes of sleep apnea. He began using oxygen at night and undertook a vigorous exercise and diet program. He shed 30 to 40 pounds and is having virtually no more apnea episodes. He feels much more refreshed and awake during the day and feels his memory is back to normal.

For many people, simple weight loss is the answer, but for others this is not enough. The obstruction of breathing continues. For these individuals, it is helpful to deliver oxygen or air under pressure through a mask fitted over the nose. This procedure, called continuous positive airway pressure or C-PAP, can be very effective. Others find it difficult to continue to use, since it is annoying to wear. Consequently, surgical procedures to open up the airway passages in the nose and throat have been developed. When these procedures were first done to treat sleep apnea, the surgeon would place a tube directly into the windpipe. These days such surgery is reserved only for extreme situations in which the sufferer has associated heart problems. Now it is more common to use radio frequency waves to remodel the tissues at the back of the tongue and around the entrance to the windpipe. This strategy opens the airway in the throat and can be done as an outpatient procedure. It causes very little pain or blood loss and so is relatively safe.

MEDICATIONS FOR SLEEP

Sleep is big business for pharmaceutical companies. Sleep complaints result in million of sales of over-the-counter sleep aids and 25 million prescriptions for stronger sleep drugs every year. Americans buy more drugs and preparations for sleeping than any other health problem, with the possible exception of headaches. Insomniacs, travelers, shift workers, and many others have long sought an ideal sleeping medication. The perfect sleep-producing drug would have several properties: It would act quickly, but not have long-lasting effects, leaving no feeling of being drowsy and lethargic the next morning. You would not develop tolerance to the drug, requiring larger and larger doses to get the same effects. You would be able to stop the drug without getting a rebound effect of insomnia. Finally, the drug would be safe. It would not interact with other common medications, and it would not be useful for people who want to commit suicide. Despite years of attempts, no such drug has been developed by the pharmaceutical industry.

In the 1960s and 1970s, the favorite drugs for sleep were barbiturates such as nembutal or seconal. These drugs had several disadvantages. The first problem was tolerance; after two to three weeks of use, it took a higher dose to get the same effect. Second, barbiturates had varying, unpredictable lengths of action. Consequently, many users woke up with a "hangover," feeling drowsy, lethargic, and depressed. Sometimes, these aftereffects led to a cycle of taking "downers" (barbiturates) at night and "uppers" (like amphetamines) in the morning. Finally, they aren't safe: an overdose of barbiturates can cause decreased breathing and death.

More recent medications included drugs such as Dalmane, hailed as a safe, nonaddicting drug. Only after wide use did it become clear that drugs like Dalmane had their own sets of problems. The drug stayed in the body for very long times—in older people evidence of a single dose could be found as long as four or five days later. Thus, after several days of use, it was not uncommon for older individuals to have problems with coordination, balance, increased falls, confusion, and depression. Accordingly, we do not feel that Dalmane should be taken by elderly people.

As a result of the problems with such drugs, the pharmaceutical companies developed drugs such as Halcion and Restoril that would clear out from the body more quickly. For a while, Halcion was the most widely prescribed sleeping medication. However, it was not the magic answer either. Many people developed tolerance to it after two or three weeks and many also had increased difficulty sleeping after the drug was discontinued, so-called rebound insomnia. Delayed effects of Halcion such as confusion, difficulties with memory, agitation, or depression also appeared after several weeks of use. These behavioral problems led British medical authorities to ban this drug at one point. However, we often recommend Halcion at a low dose (0.125 mg) for two to three days' use to overcome a short-term problem, such as jet lag.

Now, a new class of drugs for sleep has emerged. One such drug, called Ambien in the United States, appears to be short acting, with fewer side effects than Halcion and Restoril. It is currently the drug most often prescribed by doctors, but even Ambien is reported to cause confusion and memory loss in the elderly. We advise caution in its use. Another medication for sleep getting a lot of attention is melatonin. Melatonin is a naturally occurring compound made in a part of the brain called the pineal gland and normally involved in regulating our sleep-wake cycles. The evidence is quite good that melatonin can be effective in improving sleep after sleep deprivation, such as in jet lag. In addition, travelers going from west to east across several time zones take melatonin with apparent safety to prevent jet lag (one tablet each evening the five days before departure) to nudge the internal clock toward the time in the destination city. However, no such evidence exists for its long-term use for other forms of insomnia. Another possible use of melatonin is to help with rebound insomnia after someone stops taking another sleeping pill, such as Halcion. Researchers are evaluating several longer acting forms of melatonin that may be more effective than a single dose.

The FDA does not regulate the production and quality of melatonin. You can get it in any drug or health food store, yet the standards for its production can vary. We are cautious about such compounds, and advise against using melatonin on any kind of steady basis until it has been more thoroughly studied and its preparation and safety are determined and standardized.

A variety of herbal preparations list sleep as a use. Only one has been evaluated in clinical trials and shown to be effective. That is valerian, which we discussed in chapter 2, "Nutrition for the Brain: Food, Fuel, and Protection."

People in their 70s and above who are taking medications are not going to sleep a solid 8 to 10 hours per night. Attempts to induce this pattern of sleep in nursing homes are doomed to failure. In addition, people this age process medications quite differently than younger people. The dose of most sleeping medications should be cut in half for the elderly—the difference in the way it is handled by the body is that great. Failure to realize these differences can result in persons being "zonked" the better part of each morning. Perhaps it is better to recognize that older people will sometimes be awake at night and arrange for them to have books to read, a radio, television, or someone to talk to.

FUTURE SLEEP TREATMENTS

We think one of the best treatments for sleep in the future will be more health-conscious generations applying what we already know about how a healthy lifestyle can improve sleep. In short, if all of us getting older are as smart as we think we are, we'll change the things we do that might interfere with sleeping well and we'll allow enough time for sleep.

However, we do see a need for substances that can be safely taken to promote sleep on a daily basis. Worldwide, we have a "pick me up" in the morning, a cup of coffee or tea. We have no such preparation to "lie me down" at night. Perhaps some herbal preparations may fill that bill, though we need long-term studies of their safety and effectiveness. If they are shown to be effective, chemical studies should be done to identify their contents so that the elements in herbals could contribute to the development of newer sleeping medications.

WHAT YOU CAN DO ABOUT SLEEP: MAKE GOOD SLEEP A PRIORITY

Although there's no question that sleep changes as you get older, you can improve your chances of a good night's sleep by developing a sleep routine, giving bedtime the same attention and importance as the start of the day. First, establish a regular time for going to sleep and waking up. Relaxing rituals—a soothing drink, quiet reflection of the day's events, meditation or prayer, or a good book—can help, but the key word is "relaxing." If going over the day's events sends your blood pressure skyward, try a different ritual, and if you opt for a drink it shouldn't contain alcohol or caffeine. Make your environment conducive to sleep: Block morning light with curtains or a sleep mask, and try a white noise machine to mask unwanted sounds. Find the right thermostat setting or mix of bedclothes that best prevents uncomfortable temperatures.

Don't worry if your patterns for waking and sleeping have shifted a bit; they don't need to match up exactly with everyone else's. And a nap in the afternoon can be just what your body needs. But excessive sleepiness in the daytime can be dangerous, particularly if you're driving. If you or someone else notices that you sleep a lot in the daytime or you often feel very sleepy, or if your mate says that you're fitful in sleep, consult your doctor about sleep apnea or abnormal leg movements. Help is available for both of these conditions to get you back to sleep at night.

CHAPTER **4**

MANAGING STRESS

Many people considered Carol a "superwoman." In her 40s, she was the principal of a high school, the wife of a busy lawyer, the mother of three children, and somehow still found time to be involved with community activities, including the United Way and the Boy Scouts. She seemed to be able to balance all of these activities effortlessly and was well liked in the community. The first sign of trouble, in retrospect, was that she was getting very thin. Her friends began to worry that she had some underlying illness and asked how she was feeling. She responded that her stomach had been bothering her and she thought she had a stomach virus that was lingering. Finally, her husband insisted that she see her doctor.

After weeks of postponing appointments, she finally went. When medical examination showed no reason for her loss of weight, her doctor asked her if something was going on in her life that was upsetting her. After some hesitation, she began to unburden herself. The schools in her district were all going to have an outside review, right at the time that she had agreed to direct the United Way campaign. She was becoming progressively overwhelmed—she was waking up at night worrying about problems, had lost her appetite, and felt that she couldn't concentrate or get anything done. Her physician helped her recognize how much stress she was under, and encouraged her to decrease her responsibilities. After talking with her doctor, she found it easier to talk with her husband. He convinced her that it was not a sign of weakness or failure if she said "no" to requests that would add further burdens when she was already stretched to the limit. She found someone else to run the United Way campaign, delegated some responsibilities for the school review to her assistant principal, and went to the gym with her husband each weekend. Six months later, the school review was over, the United Way campaign was successful, and Carol and her family happily enjoyed a well-earned vacation.

Stress can do more than just make you edgy; it can undermine your health and possibly even speed up the aging process. Finding way to cope with stress can help you keep your mental edge, your health, and (most of the time) a reasonably good mood.

RESPONSES TO STRESS

When you are suddenly under stress, as when you have to react to a threatening or unexpected event, you develop very characteristic responses. Your brain produces substances that tell many organs of your body to speed up and perform more effectively. In response, your heart races, you become sweaty, your hands may tremble a bit, and you seem to be thinking faster and reacting more quickly. This short-term response to stress is not only normal; it is both protective and necessary. It is also short lived. When the stress is over, your body's emergency response shuts down, and things return to their normal pace.

At times like these you can sometimes handle the problem you face unusually well, being stronger and quicker than you normally are. Some people actually design their lives to keep things just stressful enough to keep themselves functioning at these higher levels. These are the people that leave preparation of a report to the last minute or do their taxes the night of April 15.

For many people, however, stress is a long-term, chronic problem. Psychologists point to major life events—loss of a loved one, divorce, loss of a job, or moving—as known triggers for longer-term stress. These are all major changes, and the accompanying problems and feelings take time to run their run course. Other long-term situations—like being the caregiver for a person with a chronic disease, or constantly worrying about money, or being trapped in an unrewarding job—may seem to offer no respite and no way out. These are predicaments that lead to chronic stress, and they take their toll.

THE EFFECT OF STRESS ON THE BRAIN

As we discussed in chapter 1, "Maintaining Your Memory," those who preserve their cognitive function as they get older also tend to maintain a degree of self-efficacy. That is, they know how to adapt to life's challenges rather than becoming overwhelmed by stressful situations. In addition, they maintain some degree of control in their daily lives and are not overly dependent on others.

We think we know why those who maintain a degree of self-efficacy are protecting their brains. There is increasing evidence that stress actually damages the brain. Research in experimental animals has shown links between severe stress and damage to the brain, particularly the brain regions associated with processing memories. The mechanism for this is thought to be the brain's response to hormones (called glucocorticoids) that increase during periods of stress. At high levels, these stress hormones can actually kill nerve cells in animals, and the same is thought to happen in humans. Thus, the steps you take to reduce stress, and, by extension, stress hormones, are likely to preserve nerve cells and thereby help maintain mental abilities.

THE EFFECT OF STRESS ON ILLNESS

Only two Americans, Greg LeMond and Lance Armstrong, have ever won the most famous and grueling bike race in the world, the Tour de France. Lance Armstrong won it not once but three times. What makes his victories particularly noteworthy is that he achieved them after he was diagnosed and treated for cancer of the testes. The treatment involved the use of anticancer drugs that weakened him and sapped his endurance. Nevertheless, he stated on numerous occasions that he was determined to overcome his cancer and get back to bike racing. After the treatments were over, it took him over a year to get back to riding a bicycle at all. No one thought he would be able to return to bike racing, let alone to the level required for the Tour de France. But he did! He believes that it was his positive attitude that made the difference. This led to his desire to establish a foundation to support and educate patients with cancer on the importance of a positive attitude.

Lance Armstrong is a very unusual example to use in a book on aging for several reasons: first he is quite young, second, he had widespread cancer but responded to therapy and was essentially cured. If that were not enough, what makes him famous is that he won the most well-known and grueling bike race in the world. None of us, in our wildest dreams, think we will do anything close to this. That does not mean we cannot learn from him.

In his book *It's Not about the Bike,* it is clear that what allowed Lance Armstrong to accomplish these feats was primarily his attitude toward what was happening to him each step along the way. He wanted to feel as if he was maintaining some degree of control over his life by becoming knowledgeable about his cancer; this enabled him to participate in the decisions about his treatment and rehabilitation. He was honest with people about what was wrong, allowing him to get emotional support from others; he acknowledges the enormous role of his mother and his coach, who pressed him to begin training again, even when his stamina was very poor.

Lance Armstrong had an unusually stressful event occur early in his life. Although most of us may not share this experience, we are all like Lance Armstrong in that we experience stress and disappointment throughout our lives. And scientists are learning that the brain and the body influence each other more than we ever thought possible. Having a positive attitude, controlling stress, and reducing depression can influence your predisposition for illness and your recovery if you do become ill.

Immune Function

The most clearly documented negative effect of chronic stress is a shutting down of the immune system, the system the body uses to fight infections and cancer. Under long-term stress, you can be more likely to get infections, even common colds. Among patients being treated for cancer, the ones who report higher levels of stress do not respond as well to their treatment regimens as those who seem to be coping better. One possible mechanism for this effect is that, in response to stress, parts of the brain release substances that circulate in the body, suppressing the immune system. The stress hormones we mentioned above (glucocorticoids) decrease the production of immune cells that are important in the body's defense against cancer.

Heart Disease

Chronic stress also increases the risk of coronary artery disease. An estimated 15 million Americans are caregivers for sick and disabled relatives (such as a child with a disabling illness or a family member with Alzheimer's or Parkinson's disease). Thus, they have often been examined as a model for studying the effects of stress. People in these situations have a greater risk not only of some of the immune changes mentioned earlier but also of both fatal and nonfatal heart attacks. However, it is not just this stress but how they respond that is important in their ultimate health.

Through his research, Guy has had personal experience with the importance of attitude and heart disease. For the last eight to ten years he has been evaluating people both before and after they have a type of heart surgery performed to deal with heart disease that causes chest pain. This procedure, called coronary artery bypass grafting, is very common: more than 400,000 people in the United States have it each year. It is done so frequently because it has the potential to make a heart patient markedly better. By being able to evaluate patients both before and after surgery, Guy has had the opportunity to determine what behavior and attitudes are associated with better or poorer results.

The patients' moods and attitudes before and shortly after surgery make a big difference in outcome. Those who have a positive attitude—who are optimistic—have fewer returns to the hospital, are less likely to have the return of chest pain, and have less need for another heart operation. In contrast, those with a negative attitude, particularly those who have symptoms of depression, either before or after surgery, are much more likely to have the return of the chest pain associated with heart disease within a few years.

It seems likely that people with a positive attitude toward illness are more motivated to participate in health-promoting activities, such as following medical regimens, being physically active, stopping smoking, and losing weight. A positive attitude may also contribute to better immune responses and better healing of wounds. Bear in mind, though, that during times of crisis such as serious illness, divorce, or death of a loved one, keeping a positive attitude may include an honest and healthy coming-to-terms with emotions often considered negative, such as grief, anger, and fear—all appropriate reactions to trouble.

How to Reduce the Effects of Stress

You can do many things to reduce stress. First, recognize that a variety of unpleasant signs may be signaling a problem. The symptoms of excessive stress can be quite nonspecific, such as difficulties with appetite, sleep, concentration, and increased irritability. Many people, like Carol, will focus on their physical complaints, not recognizing that the true cause is their response to stress.

We all live with a certain amount of stress in our lives every day. But certain situations predictably increase stress. For example, a change in marital status, a change in job status, a significant illness in a family member or oneself, or a death in the family are all high-stress life experiences and usually produce stress over long periods of time. Under these circumstances, you have to be careful about adding new potential causes of stress. Situations which, by themselves, you could handle easily may be enough to tip the balance.

Besides not adding new problems, it worthwhile to examine what you might do to change how you are leading your life, particularly when it comes to your ability to reach out to others. Many people slip into a pattern of thinking they alone can solve a problem. They have difficulty delegating to others or turning to others for help. Carol had to accept that her assistant principal would prepare for the school review differently than she would, but could still be very effective in getting the work done. She had to come to terms with the fact that everything did not have to be done by her, her way. Accepting help from others may be a key factor in keeping up your health in times of trouble. This is true even if all your friends can do is listen. One of the traits that helped Lance Armstrong was his willingness to discuss his problems.

In order to adapt to the stress of dealing with a chronic illness, it is also important to know as much as you can about the medical condition. This information can be obtained from a variety of sources, including your physician, support groups, and for the more common diseases, books or web sites are very helpful (see the Appendix). If you know what to expect, and what can be done, you can be both physically and mentally prepared.

We often discuss with caregivers the importance of taking care of themselves, of recognizing how stressful their lives have become, and of obtaining information. The worst thing for the patient would be for something to happen to his or her caregiver.

Rather than examining and changing their lifestyles, many people would rather have their physician give them a magic pill that would make everything better. Drugs to reduce anxiety and improve sleep can help, but, for most people, medications alone are not the answer.

In addition to changing some responsibilities, if possible, and taking advantage of social support, you should consider using one of the many relaxation techniques that reduce stress, such as exercise programs, meditation, biofeedback, or massage therapy.

STRESS RESEARCH

It is clear that the brain and the body interact much more, in health and disease, than we previously realized. Much of the current information is at the level of description—what we don't know are the underlying mechanisms. The effects of stress hormones on the brain and the immune system undoubtedly are only one of the mechanisms involved. In addition, there is increasing interest in how to prevent disease, and the handling of stress is likely just as important as diet and alterations of destructive behaviors, such as smoking or the use of excess alcohol.

WHAT YOU CAN DO ABOUT STRESS

Many people, particularly men, are reluctant to recognize that stress is gnawing at them and are equally reticent about talking to anyone else about their concerns. Somehow, they see this as a sign of weakness or failure. What they don't recognize is that merely talking to someone often lifts the weight, even though the source of the stress may still be present. Further, not surprisingly, they find that they are not the only person in the world who has experienced these difficulties.

For most people, developing and using social support systems is a great help in maintaining a positive attitude. By "social support systems" we mean contacts with family, friends, and organized groups including those with a religious or health orientation that have more than a passing importance in one's life. The effects of these ties can be to enhance people's perceived control of their health and over their life in general. They may also increase the likelihood that an individual will get better medical care and be more physically and mentally active.

This is particularly true when the underlying stressful situation can't be changed, as for the caregiver of a disabled family member. You can still lighten your load. Support groups do help; they provide social support and an opportunity to discuss one's feelings and to share experiences. They may do even more: some studies suggest that connections with others, including support group participants, may boost the immune system.

CHAPTER 5

Unmasking Depression

A 75-year-old widower, Eugene, had owned a gas station in the town in which he lived. He lived by himself in a small house and was well known to the shopkeepers and neighbors in his community. The owner of the local grocery store, an old fishing buddy, became concerned when Eugene didn't seem to be taking care of his personal appearance, seemed to be shopping much less often, and wasn't refilling his prescription for his blood pressure medications. The grocer called Eugene's son, who lived in a nearby city. The son first tried to reassure the grocer that his father was all right, that he was in touch with him by telephone and he sounded just fine. Eugene's son then called his father's local physician, who had known him for many years. The physician told him that his father had been to see him several times in the last year, with various complaints, particularly headaches. The physician had not been able to find any cause for the headaches and had given him some pain medicine.

Finally, at the grocer's insistence, the son came to visit. At first, he thought his father was no different than usual. He tried to get his father to talk about how he felt. That is when Eugene began to talk about his wife, who had been dead for five years. He talked about how lonely he was and how overwhelmed he felt dealing with daily responsibilities. It also became clear that Eugene had not been taking his medication for high blood pressure regularly. The son suggested that Eugene come home with him to visit, hoping that this change of scene would improve his mood. However, after about a week, it was clear that Eugene was still not his normal self. The son proposed that his own doctor meet with Eugene. The son's doctor was the first to suggest that the problem might be depression, and he urged Eugene to consult a psychiatrist. Eugene dismissed the idea that he might be depressed and certainly didn't want to see a psychiatrist. After considerable persuasion by his son, Eugene finally went as a favor to him. The psychiatrist confirmed the diagnosis of depression and started Eugene on a class of medication, then relatively new, called selective serotonin reuptake inhibitors or SSRIs, Prozac, Paxil, and Zoloft are the best-known drugs of this type.

It took about 6 weeks to bring any evidence of improvement, but, by the end of 12 weeks, Eugene was markedly better. After returning home, he took the advice of the psychiatrist and became involved with the local Chamber of Commerce, where he found needed companionship and social support.

Unfortunately, Eugene felt so much better that he stopped taking his antidepressant. Within two months his depression started to return. This time his grocer friend didn't fool around; he called the son and said, "Get down here, we've got troubles again." Eugene is now doing well, continuing on his medication. Eugene was lucky that he had a concerned friend and involved family. Persistent depression can be a life-threatening problem.

People with depression have a very poor quality of life. They are not only sad, they can become increasingly isolated due to their lack of motivation and loss of desire to interact with other people. Depression can also aggravate existing medical conditions in part, because someone who is depressed is less likely to follow a medical regimen. In Eugene's case, failing to take his blood pressure medicines put him at greater risk for heart attack and stroke.

Depression is a word we often use casually—for example, to describe that feeling of being "down in the dumps" or "blue," those times when we can't get going or are more anxious than usual or more irritable. For most of us, these are temporary changes in mood, and within several days we are back on track. But true depression is a clinical disorder, a biological disease characterized by feelings of great sadness, hopelessness, personal inadequacy, and lack of interest in things that usually capture our attention. It is also accompanied by changes in sleep or appetite.

In the past, many people viewed depression as a state of mind, assuming that someone could just "snap out of it" with a little effort. That has changed, but both the medical profession and the public have taken a long time to recognize depression as an illness. With the increased understanding have come better and better treatments. That is why today depression is considered a treatable disorder. But past prejudices die hard, and depression is still under-recognized and undertreated at all ages, but particularly in the elderly. People who might think "depression" if they saw the signs in a young person will often dismiss the same symptoms in an older person as the natural, expected response to the loss of friends or change in lifestyle. This attitude is unfortunate, because treatment can restore normal mood for many people, both middle-aged and elderly, who have become depressed.

WHO GETS DEPRESSED?

For about 3 to 5 percent of individuals in the population, the symptoms of depression are a lifelong threat. These are people who begin to be depressed when they are young and have recurring episodes of the illness throughout their life. Sometimes their depressive episodes occur every few years, sometimes only after decades have gone by. Thus, some elderly people have had depression their entire lives.

However, many elderly people get depression for the first time late in life, often with the onset of a serious medical illness. About 25 to 40 percent of elderly patients with a wide variety of diseases, such as heart attacks, kidney disease, or cancer, develop depression. Diseases of the brain, such as Parkinson's disease, stroke, and Alzheimer's disease are linked with an even higher rate of depression. Until about middle age, depression is more common in women, but, after that, the frequency is about equal in older men and women.

Depression runs in families but scientists have not yet found any specific genes for depression, despite repeated efforts by many research teams. This has led most of the researchers in the field to believe that several genes must be working in combination to increase a person's susceptibility for depression.

While the major risk for depression among older individuals is medical illness, it is not clear why this is so. Several explanations seem likely. First, quite a few common drugs can cause depression—such as medicines for the heart or for sleep—and someone who is ill is more likely to be taking multiple medications. Second, physical illness may cause changes in the body that can alter brain chemistry. Finally, general fatigue and debilitation, either of which might lead the brain to function poorly, may be enough to trigger depression. So when an older person has a serious medical illness or illnesses, it is important to be alert to the possibility of depression.

Older people are also more likely to experience bereavement and loss of stability through a change of residence, and these too bring an increased risk for depression. The fortunate thing is that the interventions, such as that we described in Eugene's case, do work for depression, regardless of the cause.

DIAGNOSING DEPRESSION

Figuring out who has depression is not always easy. For some people, the symptoms of depression may come on quite suddenly; a person may go from being functional to nonfunctional over a few weeks. The diagnosis of depression is usually easy to recognize in this instance because someone who was managing daily activities, was independent, and seemed to get pleasure from things is suddenly no longer able to do so.

However, for many older people, the slide into depression is very insidious and may go unrecognized for a long time. Even when others finally recognize it, they may find it difficult to convince this friend or relative to go for treatment. Several additional complications can hinder diagnosis when an older person becomes depressed for the first time. The elderly often do not complain about the symptoms of depression the same way that the young do. They are more likely to complain about physical symptoms, such as headaches, backaches, fatigue, and sleeplessness. It often takes a medical examination to rule out other causes and an astute clinician to recognize that these symptoms are related to depression. Another problem more common among the elderly is the difficulty of disentangling the symptoms of other serious medical illness and depression. Loss of appetite, sleeplessness, and fatigue, for example, occur in many conditions besides depression. Family members often misread the symptoms as just a part of aging. In addition, the excess use of alcohol is often associated with, and may be caused by, depression. About half the time even the patients don't suspect their symptoms might be depression.

No matter how masked the symptoms, diagnosis is important; if depression is there, it needs to be found and treated—and not just for reasons of health and quality of life. Suicide is more frequent in the elderly than any other age group, and it is the most serious risk associated with depression. It is particularly common in elderly men who are widowed. In fact, the combination of physical illness and loss of a spouse is deadly: it is the most common precipitating cause of suicide in the elderly. Sadly, many elderly people who commit suicide have talked about their intention to do so with others. In a recent study of men in their 80s who committed suicide, 70 percent had seen a physician in the previous month; one out of five had seen a doctor on the very day they killed themselves. In almost all cases, the physicians involved had neither recognized the depression nor suggested treatment. Thus, when older people talk about suicide, it is important to pay attention and get them psychiatric help.

How the Brain Is Involved in Depression

Scientists have several reasons for thinking that brain dysfunction is involved in depression. The first reason is evidence from biologically straightforward situations that shows that injury to specific parts of the brain increases the likelihood that depression will develop. People with strokes involving the front part of the brain on the left side are more likely to have depression. In addition, areas of the brain involved in emotion and memory (known as the limbic system) and parts of the brain involved in movement (including regions affected in Parkinson's disease, such as the basal ganglia) also appear to be involved. This suggests that a circuit of brain regions is important in the development of depression.

Some colleagues of ours saw a dramatically revealing example of the relationship between brain structures and depression in a woman who was having electrodes placed in her brain for the treatment of Parkinson's disease. This procedure is done under local anesthetic while the patient is awake, because the doctors need to monitor the person's ability to move and speak. To everyone's surprise, when the electrical current was applied in one particular location, the patient suddenly displayed all the symptoms of depression—she became very weepy, discussed suicide, and told everyone how unhappy her life was. When the electrical current was turned off, she rapidly returned to her normal self. This woman had no history of depression, so it was unlikely that the stimulation of her brain was arousing memories of a previous experience; rather it seems more likely that the stimulation was altering circuits in the brain involved with mood.

The other evidence for depression as a physical as well as emotional illness is that the medications for depression alter the chemistry of the brain. Very specific brain chemicals appear to be involved, primarily two neurotransmitters called norepinephrine and serotonin. It is also likely that dopamine, the neurotransmitter affected in Parkinson's disease, is related to depression. All of the medicines currently used to treat depression adjust these brain chemicals in some way. We don't know exactly what goes on in brain cells to lift depression once these medicines connect with them; we simply know these treatments work in the great majority of cases.

TREATMENT OF DEPRESSION

Once a doctor diagnoses depression, many different treatments are available. The major treatments all provide relief for older sufferers, and the approaches to treatment are varied enough to provide safe alternatives when other medical conditions are present. Some treatments, such as antidepressants, are in the category of drug therapy. This area has seen major advances in just the last few years. In addition, a modern version of the once-controversial electroconvulsive shock therapy, known as ECT, often helps in people who either cannot take medications for medical reasons or have been unresponsive to the usual medications. Talk therapy is usually used as an adjunct or follow-up to treatment with medications or ECT. Talk therapy can include psychotherapy (either individually or in groups) and family therapy (in which not only the person but also family members are involved). These forms of treatment are not mutually exclusive approaches; it is common for more than one to be used in the same person. And many people require both the continued use of medication and supportive therapy to prevent the symptoms from coming back.

Importantly, the current treatments for depression are effective in 7 to 8 out of 10 patients. That is a very high figure and is the reason why it is important to seek treatment for depression. Not many illnesses respond to treatment so effectively. Moreover, current depression treatments have many fewer side effects than they did years ago.

Medicines for Depression

Several major classes of medications are used to treat depression; all work by different mechanisms. The doctor's choice of medication takes into account several things: an individual's response to the medication, the side effects experienced by the individual, and the ease with which the medication can be taken. (Some antidepressants need be taken only once a day and some several times—depending on one's living situation, a single-dose regimen might be easier.)

All the antidepressants currently approved by the FDA are effective. The differences among them are their specific side effects and an individual's response—there is no simple answer as to what to take. The doctor may want to adjust the dosage or change the type of drug for the most effective treatment. So, the most important thing for anyone prescribed a medication is to take it as directed so that it is possible for the doctor to see how well the treatment is working.

The most common problem in treating older people for depression is undertreatment. When a person starts to take an antidepressant, the initial dose is usually at the low end of the spectrum. Sometimes a low dose is effective, but sometimes the dose needs to be gradually increased; some physicians, fearing side effects, are reluctant to try higher doses. Undertreatment may also occur when a patient tries the medication for only a short time. A fair test of an antidepressant is six to eight weeks, but many people do not realize this and stop their medication too soon, assuming it hasn't worked. A psychiatrist friend of ours says he tells his patients, "It took you a long time to get so depressed. It will take you a while to begin to feel better."

Occasionally, overtreatment is also a problem. When people who are depressed realize how bad they feel and finally go for help, they usually want a rapid improvement. They may believe that the way to get it is to take more medication. However, since higher doses of antidepressants can produce side effects, increasing the dose rapidly is likely to cause problems, convincing the sufferer that effective treatment is not possible.

The class of drug that Eugene was taking, the SSRI's, such as Prozac, Paxil, and Zoloft, have few side effects, tend not to produce the cognitive problems associated with other types of antidepressants, and are safe for your heart. For these reasons, most people who take them are more likely to stay with the prescribed routine. However, SSRI's do produce gastrointestinal upsets and impotence. Viagra can help the impotence problem in men, as we discuss in chapter 8, "Bodily Functions and Your Brain."

Another class of drugs is called tricyclic antidepressants. These affect levels of both norepinephrine and serotonin and were the standard treatments for depression for many years. Tricyclics can produce memory problems and sleepiness during the day. Unlike some of the other antidepressants, they do not affect blood pressure, but they are associated with heart rhythm problems in patients who have heart disease. Thus, cardiologists are reluctant use them.

The third type of antidepressant in current use is the MAO inhibitors (MAO stands for monoamine oxidase). Doctors seldom prescribe these medications for elderly patients because they often cause episodes of low blood pressure that can lead to falls. They also require dietary restriction (for example, you cannot eat cheese when taking them) and have more interactions with other medications. Thus, MAO inhibitors are prescribed for the elderly mostly when other antidepressants have failed.

Stubborn Cases

What if none of the weapons in this well-stocked arsenal succeeds in lifting your depression? At the end of the 1990s, new medications were introduced primarily to treat patients who did not respond to the other antidepressants. These new drugs (Remeron is one example) affect several neurotransmitter systems at once. In addition, depression treatment may sometimes succeed when another medicine is added to make the primary antidepressant more effective. The drugs that are able to provide this additive effect include medications often used to treat seizures, such as Neurontin and Tegretol.

Herbal Preparations

In Europe, the herbal preparation, St. John's wort, is widely used to treat mild to moderate depression. No studies so far have demonstrated whether the herb is more or less effective than conventional antidepressants (though one is under way). Results from the first large-scale trial in the United States, which involved 200 volunteers with major depression, showed the herb to be no more effective than a placebo (a sugar pill). At present it appears that St. John's wort might be helpful for mild depression but not for more severe depression.

If you decide to give St. John's wort a try, remember that not all preparations are the same. It is important that you use the capsules containing the extract of the plant's active substance, called hypericin. It is not entirely clear how hypericin works, but it does seem to have some MAO inhibitor activities. Even though St. John's wort is unregulated by the government, don't assume it's safe under all circumstances. It may make your skin sun-sensitive, and skin cancer is an important consideration at midlife and beyond. Some reports also suggest it interacts with other medicines, and certainly it would be a bad idea to add it to other antidepressants. We also discuss St. John's wort in chapter 2, "Nutrition for the Brain: Food, Fuel, and Protection."

How Long Should Treatment Continue?

Sometimes a person responds to the lowest dose of the first antidepressant prescribed. Other times, however, it will take different doses, different medicines, or different combinations of medicines to lift the depression. In those instances, the internist or family doctor may recommend a skilled psychiatrist to manage the changes and monitor response to treatment. Usually, when a patient is treated for depression for the first time, unless unusual circumstances exist, the doctor will have the person stop taking the medication after the depressive episode has been successfully treated. However, if the depression reoccurs, then the doctor will consider the possibility of continuing the medication throughout life. It will depend on how severe the first episode of depression was, how long it lasted, and how much it affected the patient's ability to function on daily basis.

ECT for Depression

Occasionally, medical illnesses may prevent a sufferer from taking antidepressants, or all the drugs prescribed may fail to provide relief. In these instances, electroconvulsive therapy (ECT) is a good option. The use of ECT has had a resurgence in recent years, primarily because of improvements in techniques for administering it. The thought of this treatment often frightens people because of alarming reports in the news media or dire scenarios in movies, suggesting it can damage the brain. Years ago, that might have been a risk, but ECT procedures have changed a great deal.

In electroconvulsive therapy today, the doctor places wires on the patient's head, usually on only one side. The patient receives muscle relaxing medications and general anesthesia and is not awake or aware of what is happening. An electric current then passes through the wires and produces a seizure—very fast, rhythmic signaling by the neurons—in the brain. The treatment is usually repeated three times a week for at least two weeks. It is not clear why this forceful revving up of neurons almost always reverses depression, but it is known that the seizure must be produced for it to work.

Not only is ECT both effective and safe, it has several advantages over antidepressant drugs. As we said, it can help people with medical conditions that bar using standard antidepressants, as well as people for whom antidepressants haven't worked. Another reason for using ECT is that it produces its positive effect much more quickly than medications, and, for someone who is not eating or whose depression has reached psychotic or suicidal proportions, speed is often important. Even people of very advanced age can receive ECT safely and respond effectively. Physicians have successfully treated patients up to 100 years of age using ECT.

ECT relieves depression in about 7 out of 10 cases, but its beneficial effects are often short-lived. Thus, the doctor will usually follow the treatment with a prescription for antidepressant medication, including for patients who previously either failed to respond to them or had stopped responding. Some patients for whom antidepressants hadn't worked will become responsive after ECT.

Psychotherapy and Depression

Even with the great strides in drug therapy and ECT, psychotherapy is still important in the management of depression. It helps reduce the recurrence of depression by helping develop strategies for better responding to events that tend to overwhelm the patient and precipitate depression. In this regard, psychotherapy may have particularly important benefits for elderly victims of depression, identifying and easing feelings of loneliness, abandonment, and helplessness in the face of disease. It is also helpful in reinforcing the need to stay on antidepressant medication, particularly when the medication is needed on a long-term, continuing basis.

Forms of Depression That Require Special Care

The treatments we have described don't apply to certain forms of depression. One is manic-depressive illness, a disorder that causes mood to fluctuate between depression and feelings of great elation. We often use the term "manic" to refer to someone who is very "hyper," and it is that hyper quality that is on display when a person is in the manic phase of a manic-depressive illness. Most manic-depressives begin to develop such fluctuations when they are young, but, occasionally, someone who has had several repeated episodes of depression will experience an episode of mania for the first time when they are older. In both instances, the most common treatment is lithium, a medication that appears to stabilize the mood fluctuations.

Very rarely, an older person with no prior history of depression will have a manic episode. Such a case calls for a medical evaluation, because other illnesses—for example, frontotemporal dementia (which we discuss in chapter 14, "Dealing with Alzheimer's Disease and Other Dementias")—can masquerade as mania in some people. Also rare is a psychotic depression in an older person who never had a depression earlier in life. In a psychotic depression, the individual is not only depressed but also has unusual ideas about things that are not true (such as people trying to harm them), or they hallucinate, seeing things that are not there. Again, a medical evaluation is step one, because several medications—or medical disorders, such as thyroid disease—can cause these symptoms.

IMPACT OF DEPRESSION ON OTHER DISEASES

In some situations, such as heart disease, depression appears to have a direct effect on the disease process itself. People with depression have a greater likelihood of heart attack, have a higher death rate after a heart attack, and a poorer response to coronary bypass surgery. It is not entirely clear how depression impairs recovery from medical illness. It may simply be that someone who is depressed is less likely to follow medical advice, such as taking medications, exercising for cardiac rehabilitation, and making lifestyle changes, such as stopping smoking or modifying diet.

However, some research also suggests that depression actually produces a direct physiological effect harmful to the heart, by its influence on blood pressure, heart rhythms, or the clotting of blood in the heart. Studies under way are investigating whether treating depression will improve the health of people after heart attacks.

FUTURE TREATMENTS OF DEPRESSION

The late 1990s saw major advances in the treatments for depression and progress is likely to continue well into the 2000s. New medications are always under development and the trend in the direction of greater effectiveness with ever-fewer side effects is likely to continue. Researchers are particularly emphasizing better treatments for those who are unresponsive to standard treatments. For example, they have been working on a new method of electrical stimulation that they hope might take the place of ECT. This technique, known as transcranial magnetic stimulation, sets up electrical fields in the brain by magnetic stimulation. Among its advantages over ECT, this method is simpler to use, doesn't require general anesthesia, and can home in on specific brain areas and need not involve an entire hemisphere or whole brain. In small human trials, transcranial magnetic stimulation has proved to be safe and effective. Further testing will show whether it is better than ECT.

With advances in brain imaging—scans that allow us to observe the brain working—we might also get better at determining ahead of time which of the many available treatments would be the best for an individual. For example, it seems entirely possible that we might be able to use brain imaging to predict who will respond to a particular treatment and to monitor the response to treatment.

Finally, it seems more and more clear that depression has many faces. Someone with a strong family history of depression may be very different medically from someone well past middle age who gets depression for the first time in connection with a bodily illness. Scientists are trying to sort out these variabilities on the basis of genetics, brain imaging studies, and responses to medications. Their hope is to define the specific ways that people get depression and develop well-tailored therapies for them.

WHAT YOU CAN DO ABOUT DEPRESSION: RECOGNIZE THE SIGNS

According to the National Institute of Mental Health, about 6 percent of Americans ages 65 and older have a diagnosable mood disorder, but the symptoms can be difficult to spot. Older people may not want to discuss their feelings with their doctor or anyone else and may perceive a stigma attached to mental health care. But depression is treatable, in middle-aged and elderly people as well as in young people. If you notice the following warning signs in yourself, check with your doctor; if you spot them in a friend, suggest that the person seek help.

• Feelings of guilt, worthlessness, or emptiness
• Feeling that life is not worth living
• Thoughts of suicide
• Restlessness, irritability, or anxiety
• Lack of interest in previously enjoyable activities

Depression can also masquerade under a variety of physical complaints. If you are preoccupied with any of the following, consider the possibility of a mood disorder:

• Sleeping too much or too little
• Eating too much or too little
• Headaches, stomachaches, or chronic back pain

Clinical depression is *not* a normal part of aging!

CHAPTER 6

ALCOHOL AND YOUR BRAIN

Sarah and Jim, when they were in their 40s, used to enjoy going out to dinner on a regular basis. It was not unusual for them to finish two bottles of wine or more, if another couple joined them. Now that they are in their 60s, this level of alcohol consumption rarely occurs. Part of the reason for this decrease is that they are being more health conscious—they are trying to avoid gaining weight—but they have also noticed that their tolerance for alcohol seems to have decreased significantly. Jim would not dare to drive home now after consuming one-half to two-thirds of a bottle of wine. Furthermore, if he drank that much, the next morning he would feel awful. On the other hand, his physician has told him that a little wine could actually be good for his health. He is confused about what he should do about drinking.

There is no question that moderate amounts of alcohol can improve mood by promoting feelings of happiness and reducing feelings of tension and stress—which explains the old saying, "A meal without wine is like a day without sunshine." In addition, several studies have found that, in moderation, alcohol also helps protect against diseases of the arteries of the heart. Some people, particularly the French, claim that red wine protects the heart. Whether the benefit is specifically a characteristic of red wine, or accompanies any form of alcohol, is still an unanswered question. But the good news is that the research generally agrees: moderate amounts of alcohol are good for health. Thus you can consider the limited consumption of alcohol to be healthy and safe as you get older. However, the key question when you are cruising into older age is, what is a "moderate amount" of alcohol?

DRINKING IN MODERATION

The amount of alcohol that can provide health benefits is one drink per day—and, no, you can't save up and make it seven drinks one day a week! The difficulty, of course, is that one drink seems to go "like that" and then you would like more, especially if you regularly had a couple drinks whenever you drank in your 20s and 30s. But now you have a chance to see whether you have a habit or a problem, because increasing amounts of alcohol in an older person are not good.

That one drink per day can be 12 ounces of beer (1 bottle), or 5 ounces of wine (1 glass), or 1.5 ounces of whiskey (1 shot). This may sound like very little, but as we get older, we become markedly more sensitive to alcohol. We do not absorb or metabolize alcohol any differently but we distribute it differently.

If a younger person and an older person consume the same amount of alcohol, the older person will have much higher levels of alcohol in the blood. That's because as we get older we tend to have more body fat and less muscle mass. We also have less water in our body because water does not go into fat as it does into muscle. The result is that there is a smaller volume of water in an older person to dilute the alcohol. It would be as if you added less water to a shot of whiskey: the drink would be stronger.

Even when you drink in moderation, you should be ready to take some precautions. Don't have a drink before you drive, for example. One drink for an older person leads to a higher level of alcohol in the blood and a longer time for the alcohol to clear from the body than when you were a young person. Even one drink can impair your reflex responses and judgment for several hours.

At any age, you should not take any alcohol if you are taking medications that interact with alcohol, particularly certain sleeping medications. For example, even if taken only at night for sleep, the combination of alcohol and Halcion can be lethal. Cognitive impairments from disorders such as stroke or Alzheimer's disease are also made worse by alcohol, even in moderation.

Many people take a drink at night because they think it helps them sleep. For some, however, alcohol can interfere with sleep. These people fall asleep, but do not stay asleep. In part, this is because alcohol is a diuretic and they are more likely to be awakened by the need to go to the bathroom after drinking alcohol. Alcohol also interferes with the patterns of sleep and people are less likely to fall into the deep phases of sleep needed to get a good night's rest.

THE EFFECT OF ALCOHOL ON THE BRAIN

Once you get past the one drink you can safely have, hardly an organ in the body can escape the damage that excess alcohol does, and we can't think of a disease it does not make worse. For the elderly, excess alcohol is a factor in earlier death; greater (not lesser) incidence of heart disease; more trouble with thinking, balance, and sleep; and more depression and suicide. If too much drinking continues, the brain can be irreversibly damaged. Specific areas of the brain are particularly vulnerable to alcohol—the areas involved with balance, memory, and sensation in the feet and hands. The exact mechanism by which alcohol damages the brain is not entirely clear. One of the confusing factors is that excess drinking is often associated with poor nutrition and vitamin deficiency. Thus, which part of the damage is vitamin deficiency and which part is alcohol toxicity is uncertain.

NEW LIFE, OLD HABITS

Nathan had been a successful lawyer who, after his retirement, moved to a retirement community. During his working years, he and his wife almost always had a drink or two before dinner. At his numerous professional dinners, he had done likewise. In the retirement community, he found old friends and many new acquaintances. The common greeting was, "Come on over for a drink." Soon, Nathan and his wife were having drinks at lunch and sometimes cocktails with two or three different acquaintances before dinner. After dinner, he and his wife began playing bridge, during which drinks were served.

Guy saw Nathan as a patient after Nathan had a fall in the bathroom and struck his head. While taking his medical history about why he had fallen, it became clear that the retired lawyer was going to bed every night, for want of a better word, drunk. When confronted with this, he initially denied how much he was drinking. But after a long discussion with Nathan, he finally acknowledged the amount of alcohol he was consuming every day.

Nathan never stopped drinking entirely, but he cut back to one or two drinks a night. And he turned other aspects of his life around. He became much more involved in the community, becoming a member of the board of the retirement community and chairman of their committee on finances. He is doing very well.

Several patterns of drinking in older people cause concern. A relatively small percentage has had problems with alcohol all their adult lives. More common is a pattern of gradually increasing consumption—like Nathan's.

A substantial number of people who have problems with alcohol started drinking in larger amounts in their 60s. This under-recognized problem is more common with women than with men. Women are often secret drinkers; even their children do not know that they have started drinking regularly, let alone that they have become alcoholics. This pattern of drinking has come to be known as the "hidden alcoholism" of the elderly. It is often only discovered when the elderly person seeks medical care for falls, episodes of confusion, cognitive decline, or depression. It also may be associated with abuse of other drugs, like an excess use of tranquilizers or pain medications.

Older people can be vulnerable to alcoholism for a variety of reasons, including isolation, bereavement, and depression. People who have retired or have stopped their activities due to poor health, for example, may be at special risk; they no longer have a context in which to notice their drinking problem—like having to be at work on time, to concentrate, or to be physically dexterous.

TREATMENTS FOR PROBLEMS WITH ALCOHOL

The first step in treating alcoholism is recognizing that the problem exists—by the person involved and by family members and physicians. Don't expect many alcoholics to appear at the family's or physician's door saying, "I'm drinking too much, I need help." Very often, some other problem, such as a fall or complaint of sleeplessness opens the door to inquiry for a physician.

Once an alcohol problem is recognized, the treatment for the elderly is similar to that for younger people. The predisposing social problems, such as feelings of loneliness and the difficulty of feeling sociable without a drink, need to be dealt with. Social groups to replace isolation and alcohol-free social interaction, such as in Alcoholics Anonymous, can help. For some, merely living alone *is* social isolation and is their major problem. Finding a companion or changing a living situation can be quite helpful.

FUTURE TREATMENTS FOR PROBLEMS WITH ALCOHOL

Problems with excess alcohol are actually part of a broader spectrum of addictive behaviors that include smoking, use of drugs, gambling, and even overeating. The obvious characteristic that these behaviors have in common is that, taken to an extreme, they are self-destructive.

In addition, when the behaviors are suddenly stopped, the person may have withdrawal symptoms.

Perhaps less obvious is that, unlike someone who can have a drink or play a few hands of poker and then stop, an individual addicted to any of these behaviors has an overwhelming urge to continue. We call that urge a craving. The key to medically modifying addictive behaviors is discovering the process by which craving is established and maintained in the brain. For example, if we could modify the craving of a heroin or cocaine user, something we cannot do now, we could go a long way toward solving these drug problems.

Feelings of craving involve particular regions of the brain. Evidence from brain-imaging studies shows characteristic patterns in the brain during feelings of craving. The parts of the brain important for intentionally regulating and modifying behavior are less active, while the parts of the brain involved in reinforcing behavior—memory and emotion—are more active. Even now, we depend on trial and error to devise treatments for addictive behavior. In the near future, it may be possible to use imaging of the brain to monitor whether specific treatments are returning the brain toward normal.

WHAT YOU CAN DO:
STAY ON GOOD TERMS WITH ALCOHOL

Moderate use of alcohol may be beneficial, particularly for heart disease. But moderation means just one drink (tolerance for alcohol declines measurably as one gets older). According to the National Institute on Alcohol Abuse and Alcoholism, the following are signs that a person is drinking too much:

- Drinking to calm one's nerves, forget worries, or reduce depression
- Gulping drinks down fast
- Lying or trying to hide a drinking habit
- Drinking alone more often
- Hurting oneself, or someone else, while drinking

- More than three or four episodes of drunkenness within the past year
- Needing more alcohol to get "high"
- Feeling irritable, resentful, or unreasonable when not drinking
- Medical, social, or financial problems caused by drinking

Older problem drinkers have a very good chance for recovery because once they decide to seek help, they usually stay with treatment programs. When alcohol looks like it's becoming a problem, help is easy to get from the family doctor or clergy member. The local health department, social services agency, or Alcoholics Anonymous also can help.

PART TWO

THE BRAIN AND YOUR BODY

CHAPTER 7

PAIN AND YOUR BRAIN

Sam was a coal miner in his late 50s who had crushed his foot in a mining accident. Over the next several years, the foot that had been injured became extremely painful, and his whole leg was very sensitive—he could barely touch it without setting off spasms of pain. Even the pressure of the bedclothes at night or slipping on his pants in the morning were enough to set off the pain. His solution had been to drown it in drink. When he came to see us, a young doctor working with us, a very straight-laced young man, obtained his history. When he asked, "How much do you drink?" the coal miner replied, "Sonny, I drink a lot." The young doctor, trying to be precise, suggested the largest quantity he could think of. "Do you drink six ounces of whiskey a day?" The coal miner studied the young doctor for a few moments and then replied, "Sonny, I spill that much!"

Sam was fond of his approach to controlling his pain, but he came to us because he thought we could do better. We hesitated to use opiate-like drugs for Sam, because the effects of such drugs are short-lived and he could develop a tolerance for them, requiring him to take more and more medication over time. In the end, tolerance would have increased his pain, spasms, and sensitivity.

Instead, we decided to use medications that alter the response of the connections in pain pathways. We chose to combine a drug that is commonly used to treat epilepsy, Tegretol, with a drug that was originally used as an antidepressant, Elavil. We also got Sam into psychological counseling to get his mind engaged in handling his pain and enrolled him in an exercise program to get him to use the bad leg more. The combination helped. We did not cure his pain; we modified it and helped him learn to live with it. That is often our goal for those with disabling chronic pain.

We have not seen Sam for some time, but he calls or writes every so often to tell us that his pain problem continues to be under much better control. He also reports that he "spills" less of his own medicine.

Understanding Pain

Pain occurs every day, from touching a hot stove, getting a sunburn, or twisting an ankle. But pain also may be an indication that something has gone wrong with an internal process. Stomach pain can indicate an ulcer; chest pain can be a sign of heart trouble. In these cases, pain is a positive biological force, warning and protecting us from further injury. At other times, most familiarly with chronic back pain or chronic headache, pain has a disruptive role. A system has gone awry, and pain leads to suffering and a plunge in the quality of life.

In the last 10 years scientists have made great progress in understanding the way pain works. Pain starts when tissues of the body are either damaged or distorted. In the skin, damaged tissue, such as a cut finger or sunburn, releases chemicals detected by the endings of specific nerve fibers. Other special nerve endings, such as in blood vessels, the digestive tract, or around bone, respond to being stretched. The nerves' response to stretching is the source of pain in a migraine headache, a stomachache, or in response to a broken bone. These nerves send signals to the spinal cord, and then up the spinal cord to the brain along specific pathways. In the brain, specific areas produce the conscious perception of pain; they also integrate these sensations of pain with memory and with emotional responses.

Some approaches to altering pain take advantage of particular attributes of these pain systems. Ibuprofen and similar drugs decrease the effect of the pain-associated chemicals released after tissue injury. Specific nerves carrying pain can be blocked with a local anesthetic, as a dentist does to perform a root canal. Similarly, in a procedure called epidural anesthesia, anesthetics are placed near where pain fibers enter the spinal cord. Someone who has prostate or bladder surgery has a good chance of getting this kind of pain-limiting anesthesia. Some other surgical procedures also take advantage of the specific location of pain pathways in the spinal cord and brain. The treatment for some cases of severe pain is to interrupt these pathways, either surgically or with an electrical stimulator.

Recently, researchers have discovered that the body's pain networks respond to pain in both positive and negative ways. At first the brain's pain systems tend to shut down, trying to suppress the pain. However, if pain persists, it can overwhelm these systems and they can become rearranged and may even make the pain worse. What happens is that the volleys of pain impulses coming over the nerves spread out to other nerves, increasing the signals of pain. If not treated effectively, a kind of domino effect takes hold: the pain can become more severe and more widespread. The longer the pain persists, the more difficult it is to treat effectively. This discovery is a major reason that doctors treat pain earlier and more aggressively now than in the past.

TREATMENT OF PAIN FROM SUDDEN INJURY OR SURGERY

The most common cause of pain is a sudden injury or a surgical procedure. This is true for people of all ages, but, in later years, the opportunities abound. Think teeth, snow shovels, scooping up grandchildren, or pruning the fingers along with the shrubbery. Technically, this is acute pain, and, ordinarily, it is temporary. Your challenge is to get through it as comfortably as possible; your doctor, of course, is there to help you do that.

The major change in medical management of acute pain is to treat it promptly and aggressively and not let the pain get the upper hand. The goal is to keep the pain systems from responding abnormally. In other words, the old idea of giving a painkiller after the pain got bad was wrong. Now doctors advise that you take the medication before the pain takes hold.

Surgery always damages body tissues and causes pain, but now we know that if pain medications are given during the operation, the pain after surgery ends sooner and is less intense. This change in pain management often leads to a shorter hospital stay as well. Pain treatment during surgery usually consists of using local anesthetics to block the nerves between the brain and the tissue being operated on, followed by antipain medications immediately after surgery. The success of surgery pain management has changed our thinking about treating other forms of acute or sudden pain.

Treatment for acute pain initially takes the form of a non-narcotic pain-killing drug, such as aspirin or Tylenol. Either in conjunction with these or alone, doctors also advise taking anti-inflammatory drugs, such as Motrin or Advil, at the doses recommended on the bottle. If non-narcotic drugs do not work at the maximum recommended doses, there is no point in going higher, because it will not lead to increased pain control. Doctors give these analgesics for a fairly short time because of the side effects, particularly at high doses, including nausea, vomiting, and stomach pain. Aspirin can cause stomach bleeding in some people, and should not be taken by anyone who has ever had an ulcer.

If pain persists despite these milder agents, the next step is stronger drugs, most of which are narcotics, called opiates, and include codeine, Demerol, morphine, and Fentanyl—all controlled substances that must be prescribed by a physician. With narcotics, the higher the dose, the greater the benefit. Doctors can increase the dose by either giving larger amounts or shortening the time between doses. In the past, physicians were very reluctant to increase the doses beyond a certain point for fear of addicting patients; the standard approach was to prescribe a fixed amount at specific intervals, such as every four or six hours. Now, to keep pain under control, narcotic drugs are given at shorter intervals, or even continuously. There are two ways to give the pain medications continuously. One approach is with a patch containing the pain medication that is placed on the skin. The other method is to hook up a pump with an intravenous line so that the patients can administer the drug themselves. The pump dispenses a drug such as morphine into the bloodstream with each push of the button at the bedside; the amount is preset so that the patient can't get too much medication. Pumps are used most often to treat pain after an injury or operation, either in a hospital or at home.

Many patients with cancer have pain, particularly in the terminal phase of the illness. A lot has been learned from attempts to control the pain associated with cancer. Few of these patients ever become addicted. Some, however, develop tolerance to a drug, meaning that it takes more and more medication to achieve the same effect, but opiates differ in their tendency to produce tolerance. Morphine is much more likely than Fentanyl to do so.

Treating severe pain takes some skill. Many physicians do not have experience in this area, but there are pain specialists who can outline specific pain regimens. Patients also need reassurance about management of pain. Most have been brought up to feel that the less medicine you take the better, and if you take more you will have side effects such as constipation, nausea, or confusion. They are also fed up with taking so many medications and need to be reassured that this approach will really make a difference.

Other medications besides narcotics are helpful in treating specific kinds of pain. For example, sunburn pain or that associated with a particular scourge of the elderly, shingles, responds to creams containing a local anesthetic like lidocaine. A major advance for inflammatory pain, like arthritis pain, was the discovery that a specific enzyme called a cyclo-oxygenase spurs the inflammation. The finding has led to a new class of drugs that decrease inflammation by blocking this enzyme with a substance known as a COX-2 inhibitor. Several compounds containing COX-2 inhibitors are coming on the market, including Celebrex and Vioxx. Their major advantage is that they provide pain relief with fewer gastrointestinal side effects. Since they are new, it is too soon to know if they will be safe for long-term use by people with chronic pain.

COMMON CAUSES OF RECURRING PAIN

For adults, several disorders can cause recurring pain. Back pain and headache are, by far, the most common. Recurring pain from disorders that irritate specific nerves, such as occurs with shingles, also is more common among older adults.

Each year in the United States alone, back pain, headache, pain from arthritis, and nerve pain from diseases such as diabetes, incapacitate an estimated 50 million workers. The costs of treating such pain are equally astounding, approaching 100 billion dollars with 40 million doctor visits each year.

Acute Back Strain

Guy used to see many people with complaints of back pain. Often the symptoms didn't seem to make any sense. The pain was all over the back, all sorts of movements made the pain worse, and he had to wonder how many of these complaints were psychological. Then, one day, while lifting a table, Guy felt a sudden pull in his own back. Within a few hours he could not move; any movement started spasms of pain all over the back. The next day he called a neurosurgeon, absolutely convinced that emergency surgery was indicated. An MRI of his back indicated a little wear and tear, but nothing too exciting. A day of bed rest and a little Motrin put him on the road to recovery. For all those sufferers he never quite believed over the years, this account stands as an apology.

One price humans pay for their upright posture is back trouble. Back problems are varied and often frustrating for both the sufferers and their physicians. Back pain is also very common, and if you are approaching middle age without having gone a round or two with it, you ought to be glad—though you're not out of the woods yet.

Backs are tricky structures. They "go out," to use current jargon, at the most inconvenient times. You can play tennis, lift heavy objects, and run with no problem. Then, what seems to be a simple movement, like bending over to pick up something from the floor, causes what feels like a snap in the back, and you can barely move for a few days. The problem starts as a sudden pain in the back, often not too severe. Then, after a delay, muscle spasms start; the back gets very tight and you have difficulty bending or moving. You can probably have no more helpless feeling than the apparent paralysis experienced when you are afraid to turn around or sit up because of an acute back strain. Most of the time the problem is temporary and, within a day or two, you will be much better.

We really are not sure what is going on when the back is "thrown out." Probably the facet joints, the small joints between the bones of the spine, have slipped a little. This is similar to a slippage in the joints between the two bones in a finger. When slippage occurs between bones in the spine, the pain, in turn, causes muscle spasms that can spread quite widely throughout the back.

TREATMENT OF ACUTE BACK STRAIN

Breaking up the muscle spasm is the key to recovery. That is why bed rest, massage, heat, and muscle relaxants all seem to help. Everyone has a favorite remedy for the problem of acute back pain. Some people get into a bathtub and do stretching exercises of their back while the water is as hot as they can possibly stand. One person drinks a beer, then fills the beer can with water and puts it into the freezer. Then he lies down and has his wife rub the frozen beer can up and down over his back. The mere thought of that therapeutic approach throws our backs into a spasm!

It helps to get off your feet and allow your muscles to relax a little bit. Prolonged sitting, as on an airplane or a car trip, can really make things worse, so try to be either standing or lying down. A muscle relaxant, a small dose of Valium or something similar, helps some people, as do pain medications. We prefer pain pills with anti-inflammatory properties such as Advil or Motrin.

Ruptured Discs

To understand the relationship between the spinal cord and the nerves, consider telephone poles carrying a telephone cable. From this cable, wires come off to each individual house, carrying messages back and forth. Your spinal cord and nerves are like that telephone system. The spinal cord is the cable, carrying signals to and from the brain. This cable is surrounded by a canal that is made up of the bones of the spine. Between these bones are cushions of material with soft centers, called discs. The nerves are like the wires, carrying signals to your hands and legs. These nerves leave the spinal cord and exit from the boney canal through special small openings.

The soft-centered discs between the bones of your spine act as shock absorbers when you jump or fall. Sometimes when you put sudden pressure on your neck or back, the soft material in the center of the disc explodes out of its normal position. When it does, the extruded material can put pressure on the spinal cord or on the nerves just at the point where they come out of the spinal cord. This condition is known as a herniated or ruptured disc. The neck and the lower back are the most common place that ruptured discs can occur.

An accountant in his early 50s used to unwind by competing in martial arts. After an especially active bout with a much younger man, he noticed that his left arm was quite numb. A day later he had a great deal of difficulty using that arm, and when he did, spasms of pain would shoot along the arm, particularly along the inner part toward his little finger. When examined, his doctor found his neck movements very limited; he could not twist it or bend it forward or backward at all because of pain. Any attempt to get him to use his left arm brought on shooting pain down the arm. The rest of his examination was quite normal. A MRI of his neck revealed that he had a ruptured disc. The gelatin-like material in the disc that acts as a shock absorber had leaked out and was pressing on a nerve. A course of conservative treatment was recommended—putting a harness over his neck that put pressure under his chin and the back of his head. The harness was attached to a rope that went over a pulley. At the end of the rope was a small weight of five to seven pounds. He sat in a chair twice a day for about 15 minutes and allowed the traction apparatus to put a gentle stretching pressure on the muscles of the neck. He also took some medications to relax the muscles in the affected area. This medicine also tended to keep him quieter—it is very hard to get an active person to slow down. Over the next week his arm pain eased, and he could move his neck normally. He was advised, rather strongly, that he should find some other way to get his exercise.

Treating Ruptured Discs Conservatively

Doctors usually offer two choices for a ruptured disk. One is to operate and try to remove the disc material that has leaked out; the other is a more conservative approach, bed rest—or traction, as we recommended to the accountant. Bed rest removes the forces of gravity that cause pressure between bones of the back and gives the muscle spasms time to quiet down. To confine an active person to bed, particularly if he is pain-free while lying down, sometimes it is necessary to give a very small dose of a tranquilizer, such as Valium, which also has muscle-relaxing properties.

Treating Ruptured Discs with Surgery

Trying to treat back problems without surgery is not always the right answer. Persistent pain in the face of treatment, particularly if there is evidence of increasing weakness, can force one's hand. The goal of surgery is to remove the bits of disc material pressing on a nerve. This is done through a small hole, with very little disruption of surrounding tissues. Recovery is usually rapid—within three to four days.

A neighbor, Nancy, woke up one spring morning while her husband was away, and decided that it was time to mow the grass. Their lawnmower was one of those big, heavy machines and she had not used it very often. She got it out of the garage, started it, but after a few passes, it stalled. She tried to lift the front end to clear clumps of grass, and as she lifted, she felt a sharp pain down her right leg. She could barely straighten up.

Guy got a call that afternoon saying, "I am sorry to bother you, but I'm in trouble." He went by, not quite sure what he would find. Nancy had made it to her bed, but could not move. Her whole leg hurt. When Guy lifted her right leg slightly off the mattress, the pain became much worse. Guy arranged for her to go the hospital by ambulance, and an MRI showed a large ruptured disc in her lower back, pressing on a nerve. An attempt was made to treat her with bed rest and pain medications for two to three days, but, if anything, the pain got worse. In addition, she was developing weakness of her leg. For these reasons, Guy felt surgery was the right idea. On the fourth day after the injury, she had the disc material removed. Three days later she went home without pain, but it took her about three weeks to get back to normal. Her husband bought a new, much lighter lawnmower, and, at Guy's suggestion, Nancy steadfastly refuses to learn how to start it.

Bony Disease of the Spine

As a person gets older, the bones of the spine are subjected to a lot of stresses. They respond to this by becoming deformed. When this happens, the bones themselves can press on the spinal cord or the nerves exiting from the spinal cord, causing pain. A combination of physical examination and imaging tests is used to evaluate what is going on. The presence of muscle spasm in the back, or finding weakness or difficulty walking may provide evidence of involvement of the spinal cord or nerves. It is also possible to tell if the sensations of pain, touch, or temperature are getting through the nerves correctly. Imaging techniques, such as CT or MRI scans, can show the extent to which the spinal cord or nerves are being pressed on by bony structures. Sometimes we still do a procedure, called a myelogram, which used to be much more common. In this procedure, a very small amount of water-soluble dye is injected around the spinal cord or nerves to outline them, and then a CT scan is performed to obtain a view of the relationship of the spinal cord to the bones of the spine.

SURGERY FOR BONY DISEASE

Bony disease in the neck or lower spine does not always require surgery, and, often, the pictures we get from imaging studies and the patient's symptoms are strikingly different. Many people walking around without symptoms have awful-looking backs on imaging studies. So, how does one decide on surgery? First, conservative therapy has to fail; bed rest, traction (for neck problems), and medication to relieve pain and muscle spasm do no good. The next step is to clarify the source of the pain, if possible. If there is a clear-cut abnormality on physical examination and imaging, then surgery is considered. But impatience for relief from pain is not reason enough.

A Coordinated Approach to Treatment of Back Pain

Many people who come to pain clinics have back pain, and most of them are in a group that physicians call "failed backs." The term implies that conventional medical and surgical approaches have not worked. These patients have chronic back pain but no evidence of any clear-cut abnormality; for them, surgery is not the answer. Nor are other invasive procedures such as implantation of stimulators or nerve blocks. These interventions seem to give temporary relief, but the patients then develop a whole new set of problems and fall into a cycle of repeated surgical interventions and more and more trouble. Many people who come to specialized pain treatment centers have had at least three back operations and are addicted to opiates. Their medical history often produces no clue as to why they were operated on in the first place. A colleague of ours, an excellent orthopedic surgeon, once told us, "I've seen many people incapacitated for periods of time for bad backs, but I have seen people wrecked by surgery."

If you have a chronic back problem that both conservative and surgical treatment have failed to relieve, your doctor's goal has to be to get you where we got Sam, the coal miner. That is, we didn't expect to totally remove his pain, but we knew we were going to make it better. In the past, the traditional approach by physicians was to do various diagnostic studies to try to identify the cause of the pain, to use medicines to try to relieve it, and to perform surgery if they thought it was necessary. For many patients this approach is effective, but it fails for a large number of people whose diagnostic studies do not indicate any clear-cut cause for the pain. They need a more comprehensive approach to pain management.

In the United States and elsewhere, pain treatment centers pioneered the use of integrated teams. A physician prescribes pain medicines in interaction with the other treatment regimens. A psychologist identifies the behavioral responses to pain and tries to modify them with a variety of techniques such as biofeedback, relaxation techniques, and counseling. A physical therapist works to overcome patients' tendency to stop moving their joints (or even the whole body) because movement causes pain. Joints are made to move; if they don't, they get stiff and painful when a person tries to use them. This is another vicious cycle that must be broken: pain, no movement, stiffness, and more pain. The goal of the vocational counselor is to help people get back to leading more normal lives, including resuming household activities and work. Very often the most important member of the team is the nurse specialist, who monitors how a patient is doing on a day-to-day basis, particularly the response to medications and the presence of side effects.

One of the lessons learned from the experience in these pain centers is that the pain may not be totally eliminated. It is possible, however, to reduce pain, improve physical functioning, treat mood disorders such as depression and difficulty with sleep, and to improve coping skills. Pain centers have spread throughout the country, but they are still not available to many people. However, the lessons they have provided about the integrated management of chronic pain can be used in any environment.

Acupuncture for Pain

Many people with pain become dissatisfied, or impatient, with the more conventional approaches and seek alternative methods. We subscribe to only one alternative, acupuncture, which can relieve pain when used correctly. How acupuncture helps is not clear, but it seems to bring the activity in the pain pathways back toward normal. In our experience, acupuncture is best used early in pain management; it is less likely to work for someone who has had chronic pain for many years. Many people give up on acupuncture too soon, after only one or two attempts at treatment. We recommend treatments at least two to three times a week for at least a month, because the positive effects do not all come at once. First you notice that you can do more, such as walk farther without pain, you have more energy at the end of the day, and then gradually feel less and less pain. At that point the sessions can be less frequent, until they are no longer required. The whole process may take a year. Acupuncture has another major advantage—it is safe, and virtually without side effects. However, acupuncture doesn't work for everyone, and it is not clear why.

HEADACHE

Headache is another form of pain that just seems part of the human condition. There is hardly a reader of this book who has not had a headache at some time in life. Sometimes there are clear-cut reasons, like too much to drink (the aptly described "hangover") or accompanying a cold or flu. Others have headaches when under stress. Besides these common conditions, there are specific types of headaches that physicians recognize, some of which are more common in the elderly. Most headaches involve no serious neurological disease at all and they respond to treatment with simple agents such as aspirin or ibuprofen. But others are resistant to these remedies and can be very disabling. Some headaches do mean trouble, particularly when a person has never had a headache like it in the past.

Migraine

Migraine is the most common identifiable cause of chronic headache. And there is usually a predictable sequence of symptoms. Specialists call someone with migraines a migraineur. Attaching such a lyrical French label attests to something about the fascination migraine specialists have with this disabling headache. More important, maybe, to our interest in aging, the word suggests a possibly lifelong problem, although aging often brings changes in the disorder.

In a classic attack, a migraineur will have a warning, often an interruption of vision, such as wavy lines that sweep across the field of vision. The warning, also called an aura, gives way to the headache. A migraine can be one-sided or over the whole head. It may be severe: sounds or lights become very irritating, and a migraine sufferer may have to lie down in the dark because the headache may take several hours, or even two or three days, to disappear. Nausea and vomiting often come with such attacks. Some people may have only one or two attacks a year, while others will be disabled by migraine once or twice a week. Between these attacks, a person is quite normal and without headache.

The typical migraine pattern has many variants. Some have much more striking neurological symptoms, such as weakness of one side of the body, or an acute problem with memory. Others experience temporary problems with vision or serious confusion. The same person may have several variants on different occasions.

A musically trained woman told us she normally walks around during the day with music going on inside her head. Sometimes it is classical music or popular music she knows; sometimes it is music she is composing. However, she knows she is going to have one of her migraine headaches when all this internal music stops. In addition, the sound of actual music becomes very disagreeable to her. She had recently started hormone replacement therapy with a regimen that included progesterone. While on that regimen, her migraine attacks became both more frequent and more severe. During this time she attended a concert she had been looking forward to for some time, but she had to leave at the intermission because she found the sound of the music so unpleasant. Changing her hormone replacement markedly reduced the severity of her attacks. Between migraine headaches she is now her usual musically inclined self.

Sometimes people have neurological symptoms but no accompanying headache. Specialists call these episodes "migraine equivalents." For example, children sometimes have temporary episodes of abdominal pain ("abdominal migraine") or cycles of vomiting that many physicians would consider migraine, primarily when the child's family has a strong history of migraine. Adults may have symptoms such as weakness of one side of the body, numbness of a leg, or temporary decrease in vision, but not headaches. When we see such a patient, we attribute their symptoms to migraine, rather than some other disorder, because they have had similar symptoms along with migraine in the past.

As people get older, their migraine headaches may change. In the most common pattern, they have classic migraine attacks through their 30s and 40s, and then the headaches disappear for many years. They may then return when people reach their 60s or 70s, but be different. Often, the aura may not reappear, just the headache. Some people have the reverse, just the auras, but no headaches.

Who Gets Migraine?

Migraine can begin at any age, though only about 1 in 10 migraine sufferers is a child. Migraine is more common in women. In the general population, about 6 percent of men, and 20 percent of women report having migraine. Some have said that intelligent women are particularly susceptible, others have singled out compulsive men. At least half of patients with migraine have close relatives who also have migraine headaches. Consequently, researchers are tremendously interested in the genetics of migraine. Recently a rare form of migraine, headaches associated with weakness of one side of the body, has been linked to a specific genetic defect. The gene regulates how cells respond to one of their signaling components, the ion, calcium. This new genetic information could prove to be the forerunner to getting at the genetics of the more common forms.

What Triggers Migraine?

Many triggers can set off episodes of migraine: alcohol, stress, menstruation, certain foods (particularly chocolate, cheeses, and wine, most often red wine), and medications such as estrogens or progesterone in women. An interesting and not uncommon phenomenon is weekend migraine, suffered by people only on weekends, when they try to relax.

Hal had a history of migraine attacks about four or five times a year. He had been perfectly fine until, after working hard all week, he took a nap late one Saturday afternoon in preparation for a dinner out. His wife noted that he seemed very confused when he woke up. As he started to drive to their friends' house for dinner, he didn't seem to know where he was going. His wife took over the driving, and it became apparent that he didn't remember what they had done that morning. In the emergency room an hour or two later, he had almost no ability to take in new information and retain it. When asked to remember and recite the names of three objects in the room, he had a great deal of difficulty. He had gone to a lacrosse game a week before, but he had no recollection of going to that game, who had played, or who had won. He was unsure of who was president of the United States and who had recently been president. About six hours after the start of his confusion, he began to have one of his typical migraine headaches. His confusion cleared up after about 48 hours, but he was left with a permanent gap in memory. He is now otherwise quite normal.

Sorting out what causes attacks can be like solving a detective story. One thing that helps is keeping a headache diary, listing not only the headaches but also their characteristics, when they occurred and what you were doing or eating before an attack. Eventually, patterns may emerge that can lead to helpful behavior or diet modifications.

What Are the Mechanisms of Migraine?

Doctors used to think migraine was related to problems with the blood vessels in the brain and the dilatation of blood vessels in the scalp. Many people with migraine have noticed that, while they are having a headache, the blood vessels on the side of their heads are swollen and tender. The neurological symptoms, on the other hand, were thought to be from constriction of blood vessels.

Recent evidence, from imaging studies of patients during attacks and patients' responses to particular medications, suggests that abnormalities of function of blood vessels are not the whole story. Rather, abnormally functioning nerve cells release chemicals that irritate blood vessels, causing pain. These changes in nerve cells account for other symptoms besides pain, such as changes in mood, memory, and concentration. The aura, visual changes such as wavy lines that the sufferer often sees before the headache phase of migraine, are probably caused by alterations in nerve signals in the area of the brain involved with vision. The discovery that the neurotransmitter, serotonin, is involved in these alterations in nerve function has brought major advances in treatment of migraine in the form of drugs that modify the actions of this neurotransmitter.

TREATMENT FOR MIGRAINE

Migraine treatment consists of prevention, nondrug treatment, treatment of the acute symptoms, and long-term treatment. Prevention involves figuring out what triggers attacks, using a diary as outlined above. We have a diet list we give patients that notes the foods that commonly precipitate attacks. The foods we most often warn people about include chocolate and red wine. After that, we may need a lot of trial and error to pinpoint what causes trouble in a particular person.

Many people reduce the number of their migraine episodes by modifying their behavior, for example, by reducing stress. Some people learn on their own how to do this; others find techniques such as biofeedback or psychological counseling helpful.

For acute migraine, treatment starts with simple medications like aspirin or Tylenol and then goes on from there. A drug often added is ergotamine in one of its several forms (such as Gynergen), a medication first used in the 1930s that must be taken at the onset of an attack to be effective. One of ergotamine's actions is to narrow the blood vessels in the affected area, but it may also work by modifying the neurotransmitter, serotonin.

Recently a class of drugs originally used to treat heart pain has proved successful in treating complicated migraine. These agents, called calcium channel blockers, modify how calcium binds to blood vessels. In this country Verapamil is now used. In Europe, Fluorapin, a similar agent, is widely used.

The newest drugs act like serotonin and bind to specific receptors on blood vessels and nerve cells, bringing their function back to normal. The first, Sumatriptan, which came on the market in the late 1980s, originally had to be given by injection, but is now available in an oral form, as a nasal spray, or as a suppository. Sumatriptan can be successful in reducing migraine attacks about 70 percent of the time. It relieves not only the headache but also the associated migraine symptoms like nausea or intolerance of lights and sounds. Not surprisingly, other compounds soon appeared with names like Zolmitriptan, Naratriptan, Rizatriptan, or Eletriptan. They are all very similar drugs, and some work faster than others. One person may respond better to one than another, so the physician sometimes has to try several before finding the best one for a particular patient.

Some patients have such frequent migraine attacks that some form of long-term medication is required. Most longer acting agents, such as a drug called Sansert, also work by modifying serotonin. These preventive drugs are used cautiously because they have potential side effects, particularly on the heart, that require careful monitoring.

Other Types of Headaches

Headaches come in many varieties, and each has a slightly different treatment.

CLUSTER HEADACHES

Cluster headaches are first cousins to migraine. Like migraine, they can come on in middle age and worsen progressively as one gets older. They come in bunches, one to three attacks a day for four to six weeks; they then subside for weeks or months. The headaches can be seasonal, perhaps occurring every spring. Cluster headaches are almost always on only one side and can be very severe. The biology of cluster headaches is probably similar to migraine, because they respond to similar treatment.

TENSION HEADACHES

Tension headaches start in the muscles, arising particularly from muscles in the back of the neck and scalp. They are associated with stress, eye strain, poor posture, and fatigue. Classically, tension headaches develop as the day progresses and reach their peak toward the end of the day. Anyone who spends a good part of the day staring at a computer screen is well aware of this type of headache. Mild painkillers, like Motrin or Tylenol, stretching the muscles involved, and avoiding maintaining the same position for long periods of time can all help to lessen these headaches. As with migraine, a headache diary can help to define the triggers for the headache.

Long-term tension-type headaches often come with stress and anxiety. Their proper management depends on recognizing these outriders and modifying them with anti-anxiety and antidepressant medications. Continued use of painkillers, alone, will not be effective.

HEADACHES WITH ILLNESS

Some illnesses that occur more often in the elderly cause headaches. Diseases of blood vessels, lungs, and bones can all be an underlying cause. Medications for these conditions can also contribute to headaches, as can other diseases.

HEADACHES FROM INFLAMMATION OF BLOOD VESSELS

The source of these headaches has an odd name, giant cell arteritis, a condition in which arteries develop an inflammation, an allergic reaction with swelling and immune cells infiltrating the artery walls. Why this inflammation happens is a mystery but it occurs almost exclusively in the elderly, being 10 times more frequent in people in their 80s than in people in their 50s. Giant cell arteritis is a generalized disease with aches of the muscles and joints and fatigue, but headaches are the most common early symptom. The headaches get progressively worse, and the scalp may become very tender to the touch, particularly along the sides of the head. Sometimes the arteries in this region are swollen and very painful. A bad complication occurs when the arteries of the back of the eye, the retina, become involved: it can lead to loss of vision. Doctors can diagnose the disease from its symptoms, but the diagnosis is confirmed in two ways: taking a small piece of a scalp artery and looking for the inflammation under the microscope, or by a blood test, called a sed rate, that measures the process of inflammation.

Giant cell arteritis is very treatable, but untreated it can cause blindness and strokes. The drug, Prednisone, a form of steroid hormone, makes the symptoms disappear like magic. However, the condition is a chronic one, and people may have to be on low doses of Prednisone for months, if not years.

HEADACHES WITH LUNG DISEASE

As people get older, some develop the chronic lung disease called emphysema, in which they do not move air in and out efficiently. These same people can get headaches, probably because they accumulate too much carbon dioxide, the gas that the lungs normally remove. The headaches are usually present in the morning, and get better when the person is up and about. Relieving the lung disease removes the headaches.

HEADACHES FROM MEDICATIONS

Almost any medication, from drugs for blood pressure to those for pain—including over-the-counter and alternative preparations—can cause headaches in some people. Coffee and alcohol also can be the problem. In seeing someone with headaches, after we make sure the headaches are not related to disease, we start to suspect medications, particularly newly added medications.

SUDDEN UNCOMMON SEVERE HEADACHES

If a person has a long-standing history of headaches, or previously had migraines, we worry less about a serious underlying problem. We do become concerned when a patient comes in with a headache who has never had one like it before, or complains of being awakened by early morning headaches with associated symptoms such as nausea, a stiff neck, fever, or changes in behavior or neurological functioning. In an elderly person with a new headache, we try hard to find a cause.

When a person walks into an emergency room saying, "I have the worst headache I've ever had; the top of my head is blowing off," the attending physician should be thinking, "Look out, this could be trouble." This person might have a burst blood vessel or an acute infection. Simple screening tests, such as imaging with a CT scan or MRI, which can detect blood, or a lumbar puncture, which can find evidence of infection, are standard practices in an emergency room.

HEADACHES WITH BRAIN TUMORS

When many people go to the physician complaining of headache, their secret fear is that they have a brain tumor. The truth is that of every 1,000 people complaining of headaches, fewer than one has a brain tumor as the underlying cause. But for older people, brain tumors are more frequent, so our suspicions are aroused when the headache is a new occurrence or different from previous headaches. Brain imaging is so safe, quick, and reliable, that it is very easy to allay someone's concerns. Medicare and most other insurance carriers cover these diagnostic tests.

PAIN THAT COMES ON WITH INCREASING AGE

While you are odds-on to someday have one of the pain problems already discussed, certain types of pain increase markedly in late midlife and old age. The reason for this predilection for the elderly is unclear.

Shingles

Shingles occurs in older people who had chicken pox many years before, usually in childhood, and is a peculiar manifestation of the same infectious agent, the chicken pox virus, Herpes Zoster. The virus lies dormant for many years in nerve cells. For reasons we have not yet figured out, 60, 70, or even 80 years later the virus wakes up in 1 or 2 nerves of the trunk or face.

The first symptom is usually a band of skin rash that runs across the back around to the front or over one side of the face and resembles the rash of chicken pox, with small bubbles (called vesicles). Pain and itching may come before the rash, but for people 60 and older that is not the main problem. As the rash heals, pain often persists in the involved area—a very disagreeable sensation, often a constant throbbing or burning and an intermittent stabbing or shooting pain. The pain may be made worse by touching the skin or even the friction of clothing against the skin and may go on for weeks, months, or even years. The pain of shingles can be very debilitating, causing sleeplessness, loss of appetite, and depression. It is difficult to describe how miserable a person with shingles can feel. This may be because previously they were quite well, and then "bam," they are disabled with pain.

In people younger than 40 or 50, shingles is more likely to occur if someone has immune system abnormalities, such as happens with AIDS, is receiving chemotherapy for cancer, or is taking high doses of steroids, such as cortisone. However, older people don't need any predisposing problems; shingles just happens. As mentioned above, the likelihood that the pain will persist after the acute rash is much greater in older people. So, as our "Baby Boom" generation gets older, we can expect to see more cases of pain related to shingles.

TREATMENT OF SHINGLES

No one should fool around with shingles, expecting to ride it out. Shingles needs to be treated early—and aggressively. We first treat the viral infection with antiviral drugs such as Acyclovir or similar agents. These antiviral agents have to be given promptly to do any good. The goal is to stop the virus's activity before it damages the nerves and pain becomes established.

Once the pain appears, it is important to try to bring it under control quickly because antiviral agents do not help the long-term pain. Creams containing an anesthetic such as lidocaine or a substance made from peppers, capsaicin, can help. The physician might also want the patient to take one of the drugs often used to treat epilepsy, such as Neurontin. These drugs may be more effective if started early, at the first appearance of the rash and pain. As in other forms of chronic pain, drugs used for depression, like Elavil, can help relieve the pain. In severe, long-standing pain from shingles, a morphine pump may be necessary to administer the drug.

A new vaccine can now prevent chickenpox in children. However, research suggests that the modified virus in the vaccine can still hide in nerves for many years, just like the natural chickenpox virus. Because the interval between childhood chickenpox and shingles in the adult is so long, sometimes 70 to 80 years, it will take a long time to figure out if this vaccine ultimately prevents shingles. Trials going on now are investigating whether giving the vaccine to adults will boost the immune system so that the virus will not escape and produce shingles.

Pain over the Face

Trigeminal neuralgia or tic douloureux is sharp, stabbing pain over the face, in one of the branches of the trigeminal nerve, which provides sensation to the face. The spasms of pain are induced by touching trigger points that are often over the gums or inside the cheek. A person may have trouble brushing his teeth or drinking a cold liquid. Not uncommonly, a sufferer who does not realize what the pain is will seek dental help and have needless extractions of teeth and other useless treatments.

We do not know exactly what causes tic douloureux. Most theories, but no proof, blame chronic infection of the nerve by a virus. While viruses can exist in a latent, or resting, form in nerve tissues, it is hard to prove that these viruses cause disease. Tic douloureux, like shingles, is much more common in the elderly.

TREATMENT OF PAIN OVER THE FACE

A physician colleague of ours in his 70s has this problem. He calls the pain "jabs." It occurs over his right cheek and under his right eye. Touching the upper gums on the right side of his mouth will send him into orbit. When his jabs are strong, they will take his breath away, stopping his speech in mid-sentence. For several years, he kept the pain under control by taking a medication called Tegratol. However, the beneficial effect began to wear off and he had to take more and more to get the same level of relief. On these higher dosages, he felt "dopey" and sought some other treatment. A neurosurgeon used an electric current to partially destroy the nerve supplying his face. Though his face is now numb, he is free of pain.

Pain over the face from trigeminal neuralgia is helped enormously by Tegretol, a drug for seizures. It can often clear the symptoms completely, but occasionally the response only lasts for a few months. If the pain recurs, simple surgical procedures can relieve the pain. Until recently, neurosurgeons used an electric current, as was done for our physician friend. Now a less invasive procedure, a focused irradiation known as the gamma knife, is used. A problem after such surgery is that the skin of the cheek associated with the blocked nerve is numb, and it can take a while to become accustomed to the numbness. Also, these damaged nerves do grow back, and after a few years the pain can recur. If this happens, a second nerve block can provide relief. Most people who have this treatment wonder why they waited so long.

Pain in the Feet

As a person gets older, the ability of the nerves to send signals to the spinal cord and to the brain gradually decreases. For some people, this loss of sensation can be severe and be accompanied by pain and discomfort—often a burning sensation, particularly at night, that is quite disagreeable. This problem is particularly common in those with diabetes, but, in many patients Guy sees, try as he can, he cannot identify an underlying cause. The search involves many kinds of methods, including nerve conduction studies to tell us if the nerves are sending signals correctly and biopsies of the nerve and skin to see what is wrong. Recently physicians have been using a method of skin biopsy that requires only a tiny piece of skin. Then with special dyes, the physician can tell the status of the nerves that supply the skin.

A person with pain in the feet should be patient with the doctor. The treatment of pain from abnormal nerves requires trial and error. Here again, new medicines have been helpful, particularly some first developed as anti-epilepsy drugs, the best of which is Neurontin. Physicians also use antidepressants and anesthetic creams, as is done with shingles. When a pain is severe, a cream containing capsaicin, made from hot peppers, can help by damaging the pain fibers even more, so they cannot send messages of pain up the nerves to the brain.

Someone with poor sensation in the feet has to be very careful to avoid injury. Blisters, splinters, and even burns can go unnoticed. If the injury gets infected, it can cause real trouble. Guy advises patients with this problem not to go barefoot. It is too easy to stub toes or burn feet on hot sand or hot pavement, without realizing it. It is important to look at the feet and see if there is any injury. (Sometimes, when vision or movement is restricted, this inspection is better done by a spouse or partner.) Any injury should be treated with a local antibiotic such as Bacitracin ointment. Also, Medicare covers visits to a podiatrist (foot doctor) for regular checkups.

Pain Associated with Cancer

In some circumstances, a patient's pain remains extremely severe despite the usual medications. Difficult situations, such as the person with cancer involving bone, justify extreme approaches. Many of these patients may have a limited life expectancy, so the goal is to keep them as comfortable as possible during their remaining time. In the past, physicians were too timid in their approaches. Now they treat cancer pain very vigorously, using as high a dosage of narcotic medication as necessary, until the side effects become the limiting factor. Pumps for self-administration of narcotics were first developed to control pain from cancer. One approach used only in extreme situations is to place opiate-like drugs directly into the brain. Since the drug is going directly to the parts of the brain that control pain, relatively low amounts can provide pain relief with fewer side effects.

Another way to treat severe pain from cancer does not actually require drugs; it involves the direct electrical stimulation of the brain. Electrodes are placed in the areas of the brain where pain fibers make connections on their way up to the cerebral cortex, the "thinking" part of the brain. When the current is turned on, it interrupts the incoming pathways carrying pain signals. Thus, even though the fibers from the source of the pain are firing, the part of the brain that recognizes and reacts to the pain is not getting the messages and does not "feel" the pain. We used to interrupt these pathways with surgery, but nowadays brain stimulators are used.

The bottom line of these various approaches is that there is no reason for a person to die in pain.

NEW APPROACHES FOR TREATMENT OF PAIN

Pain treatment is an enormously active area of research. Newer approaches to handling pain are in the works for all the levels of the nervous system where pain is processed. These include the site of injury, the pathways in the spinal cord that send pain messages to the brain, and the brain centers that process pain signals.

Blocking Pain at the Site of Injury

A cut finger hurts first at the site of the cut skin, because the nerves that carry pain are damaged. After the bleeding stops, the nerves are relatively quiet for an hour or so; then the whole finger becomes very sensitive to touch. If you experiment by poking around the cut a little bit, you will find that the area right over the cut is sensitive, as you would expect. However, if you move off to the edge, maybe a quarter or half an inch away from the cut, that seems to be very sensitive, too. This greater sensitivity develops because the damaged tissue has released chemicals that make surrounding nerves more sensitive to pain.

One of the hottest areas in pain research is understanding how pain fibers respond to chemicals released by injured tissue that cause pain. Scientists have discovered specific receptors in nerve cells that bond with pain-inducing chemicals and are now trying to develop substances that block these receptors. If they can do it, that would nip pain in the bud: The initial pain signal would not be turned on. So, if one had a burn, the skin would be damaged, but the pain would be much less. Imagine having a pill or spray around the house to use immediately after an injury occurs. You could even take a shot of this magic preparation before going to the dentist!

The discoveries we make about what happens at the level of the skin have implications for migraine. The chemicals released by abnormally firing nerve cells that irritate blood vessels to cause pain may be similar to those in the skin. Thus, substances developed to block pain fibers in the skin may also be used to block pain fibers on blood vessels that cause migraine.

Changing the Response to Pain

Pain signals first reach the brain as sensory information—"tissue torn," for example. But then the signals go on to check in with the emotional and memory centers—"we hate this" and "we suffered this same pain the last time you lifted that couch." The longer pain goes on, the more likely it is that pain will start to involve these other parts of the brain. This is how pain becomes chronic, but we know very little in detail about how these key steps work in pain processing. Research using the newer forms of imaging to analyze pain responses will likely shed some light on these mechanisms. Perhaps we will find that modifying the associations of mood and memory from pain can mitigate chronic pain.

Suppression of Pain

A person can have an amazing ability to ignore pain under certain circumstances. This is common in athletes during competition. A competitor may break a finger or a hand and still continue playing. The next day, he or she feels the pain just as anybody would. How is this possible? Scientists believe it is because the brain makes its own chemicals, called endorphins, that act like opiate drugs to modify pain. Some endorphins are 50 times more potent than morphine, and it seems likely that your brain uses its endorphins to modify your responses to pain. So far, it has not been possible to harness this response to pain, to turn it off and on, but many scientists are trying to see if it can be done. It would be helpful in circumstances when pain is predictable, such as surgery.

WHAT YOU CAN DO ABOUT PAIN: ASK FOR THE HELP YOU NEED

Many people in pain suffer needlessly. Older people in particular may be reluctant to speak up, perhaps because they don't want to be a problem or perhaps because they value self-reliance and stoicism. The problem of pain in the elderly often goes unremarked by family and even doctors, partly because of the unfortunate assumption that pain is inevitable as a person ages. This is not true; most pain conditions can be treated. If you are suffering, get help.

The American Pain Foundation publishes a *Pain Action Guide* that starts off with a patient's bill of rights. These rights include:

- The right to have your report of pain taken seriously and to be treated with dignity and respect by doctors, nurses, pharmacists, and other health care professionals.
- The right to have your pain thoroughly assessed and promptly treated.
- The right to be informed by your doctor about what may be causing your pain, possible treatments, and the benefits, risks, and costs of each.

Admitting that you are in pain is not a sign of moral weakness, so ask your doctor for treatment. Because pain is subjective—it isn't something the doctor can test for—be specific when you describe it. For example, rate the intensity of the pain on a scale of 1 to 10. Use specific words, like "burning," "stabbing," or "aching." Keep track of where in your body the pain occurs, what time of day it's at its worst, and whether physical activity makes it better or worse. If your regular physician is not trained in pain management (and many are not), consider seeing a pain specialist. Ask for a referral or check with an advocacy group such as the American Chronic Pain Foundation. See the Appendix for more details.

CHAPTER 8

BODY FUNCTIONS AND YOUR BRAIN

Tim had every reason to be pleased with his success navigating middle age: he sprinted from his 50s into his 60s at full stride, and, though he had developed high blood pressure and diabetes, he had a pretty good handle on both. But, on a visit to his doctor he mentioned, out of the blue, that he had been impotent (unable to achieve and maintain an erection) for the last three years. At first, he said, he and his wife joked about it, calling his blood pressure medicine his "no-go pills." But as time went on, it was no longer a joke.

At the time, a new medicine, Viagra, was just coming on the market. His physician had never used it, but he and Tim decided to experiment. The results were spectacular—Tim began having sex with his wife at least twice a week. Neither he nor his wife had realized what a psychological burden his impotence had been until it was corrected.

Despite all the fascination with sex in our culture, nobody much cared to talk about or study sex in older people, until recently. Many physicians who wouldn't hesitate to discuss the effect of a medication on sexual function with a man in his 30s or 40s didn't even bring up the subject with older men. A myth has reigned that somehow aging and sexual dysfunction are inexorably linked. That myth is wrong. Another area that patients often do not discuss with their physicians is problems with urination. These two functions, sex and urination, do change with age, but there are things that you can do about it. The topic may seem a strange one in a book about the brain, but the brain is a controlling force of these functions.

Now that researchers are at last studying sex among seniors, they are learning the truth: Men and women in their 70s don't differ very much from those in their 50s in terms of their sexual activity. If both members of a couple are in average health, sexual activity often continues and is enjoyed by both men and women. Among couples between 60 and 75, about a third have sexual activity at least once a week, and, more significantly, they report that sex is important to them. One problem women have is that their longer life expectancy leaves them without available partners. It seems that one good way to solve the sexual problems of older women would be to produce more 75-year-old men.

PROBLEMS OF SEXUAL ACTIVITY IN MEN

Men have a gradual decrease in the hormone testosterone starting about age 50, a drop that might be associated with a decrease in overall muscle mass and strength. Studies have turned up no conclusive evidence tying age-related decreases in testosterone to changes in sexual desire or performance. That is why doctors don't recommend testosterone replacement therapy for normally aging men, especially since research does show a possible link between testosterone and an increased risk of prostate cancer.

However, difficulty in achieving or maintaining an erection (so-called erectile dysfunction or ED) does increase with age, because illnesses that are more common as people get older (and the drugs prescribed for those illnesses) cause ED. In men under 65, impotence occurs about one in four men, whereas in those over 75 it occurs in about one in two men. ED has many causes. Medications are the culprit in about 25 percent of the cases. The new medications for depression, such as Zoloft and Prozac, have a particular impact on erectile function, as do many drugs used for high blood pressure. Other common age-related conditions hamper erectile function, particularly diabetes and the effects of surgery for prostate cancer. However, newer prostate surgeries, the so-called nerve-sparing procedures, have decreased the problem of erectile dysfunction in the aftermath. Psychological problems can cause ED, but older men get a break here: mental blocks are much more likely to cause the problem in younger, rather than older, men. Alcohol may lower inhibitions, but it can also knock out the ability to perform.

Treatment of Sexual Problems in Men

In 1998, the drug Viagra appeared on the scene, taking ED out of the closet. Viagra has turned out to be an amazingly effective form of treatment, returning 7 out of 10 men to near normal sexual function, regardless of the reason for the erectile problems. Viagra is particularly effective when the underlying cause is diabetes or medications. Somewhat surprisingly, even if the cause of erectile problems is damage to nerves—for example, from surgery or radiation for prostate cancer—Viagra may still be effective in about half the people. Many urologists feel that Viagra should be tried in all men with erectile dysfunction, unless medical reasons, such as heart disease, preclude it.

Viagra is a pill; the dose for elderly men is 25 mg and up to 100 mg in younger men. It takes about an hour to kick into action and is effective for about three to four hours, making the penis respond better to touch during that time. Viagra's major side effects are headache (which about one in four users experience), blurring of vision, upset stomach, and a stuffy nose. A lot of publicity has surrounded cases of men who have had heart attacks, or even died, while having sex while using Viagra. If you happen to take a particular class of heart drugs, called nitrates, you should not take Viagra, because the combination can result in dramatic drops in blood pressure leading to fainting or not enough blood to the heart or brain. For any man, your underlying physical condition matters. A person with heart disease would not go out and immediately try to run a 100-yard dash. The same is true with sexual activity. Use a little common sense, and don't try to make up for months or years of failure of sexual function with the first dose of Viagra.

One final note of caution: Viagra first appeared on the scene in 1996 and was approved for marketing in 1998; thus, its track record doesn't include long-term experience with its use. Some short-term statistics are available. After one year of use, almost 9 out of 10 men to whom Viagra was prescribed were still using it. For now, at least, it appears to be safe. Nobody knows if safety concerns will appear for men who have used it much longer. Viagra already has competitors, and there will be more. One challenge is to design a drug that acts more quickly. Viagra's maker has studies under way with forms of the drug that would be more rapidly absorbed, such as a nasal spray or a wafer that could be placed under the tongue, but these ideas are still in early exploration.

PROBLEMS OF SEXUAL ACTIVITY IN WOMEN

Women have major hormonal changes associated with menopause, one of which is a marked decrease in estrogen. For sexual function, the major impact of the estrogen decrease is a vaginal dryness that leads to discomfort during sexual activity. Estrogen replacement through pills or creams will restore vaginal lubrication. Many women also report decreased sexual drive following menopause.

Treatment of Sexual Problems in Women

A combination of estrogen-androgen replacement can improve sexual desire, satisfaction, and frequency. It is important to note that estrogen replacement has other effects, both potentially positive and negative. One demonstrated benefit is a reduced likelihood of developing osteoporosis. Long-held hopes that estrogen replacement would reduce women's heart disease began to flicker when a large study confirmed the reports of several smaller studies that replacement did not protect women who already had signs of coronary artery problems. Studies are still going on to determine whether estrogen replacement might be protective before any heart disease develops. Likewise, there are studies examining whether estrogen replacement might reduce the likelihood of developing Alzheimer's disease (see chapter 14, "Dealing with Alzheimer's Disease and Other Dementias"). On the other hand, as we discussed previously, some women appear to have an increased risk of breast cancer with estrogen therapy, particularly those with a family history of breast cancer. Therefore, we recommend that you very carefully discuss with your doctor any decision about using hormone replacement.

Many of the medical causes of decreased sexual function in women are similar to those described for men above. As with men, women who take the newer antidepressant medications have decreased sexual responsiveness. Viagra appears to be able to treat this in women as in men. Surgical procedures, such as a hysterectomy, can damage nerves in women, just as prostate surgery can do in men. Viagra increases the blood flow to the clitoris and vagina in women, just as it does to the penis in men. It is not marketed for use in women, so most of the results of improved sexual function in women are anecdotal. There are organized studies in progress regarding the use of Viagra in women, but the results are not yet available.

THE SEXUAL RESPONSE

Researchers divide the sexual response into three phases: desire, excitement, and orgasm. The brain and spinal cord are involved in all three.

Sexual desire works through the part of the brain called the hypothalamus. Injury in this area, such as from a tumor, can markedly reduce sexual desire. You can think of this part of the brain as a kind of control center, through which other parts of the brain exert their influences. For example, if you watch an erotic video, or think erotic thoughts, the vision and thinking parts of your brain are involved and send their messages through the hypothalamus. The hypothalamus then sends signals down the spinal cord to nerves that change the blood flow to the genitals. The areas of your brain just behind your forehead, the frontal lobes, discipline sexual behavior, primarily by inhibiting inappropriate responses, such as pouncing on your mate in the grocery store. If your frontal lobe control is diminished, temporarily as by alcohol or more permanently by a progressive neurological disease, this control may be lost and may result in inappropriate sexual behavior.

The excitement phase of sexual arousal may start with mental stimulation, but sensory stimulation to the penis of a man or the clitoris and vagina of a woman can also bring it about. These parts of the body have a very dense supply of nerve endings and are very sensitive to touch and other stimulation. Arousal is marked by increases in blood flow to the genitals in both men and women. In men, arousal causes erection of the penis; women experience expansion of the clitoris and changes in the shape and lubrication of the vagina. These arousal changes are a reflex action orchestrated by nerves from the spinal cord sending messages to the blood vessels and chambers of the genitalia. The common reason for male impotence and changes in responses in women is a failure of these signals from the nerves and/or the failure of the blood vessels to respond. Viagra works by strengthening the nerve signals to blood vessels and making them last longer.

Orgasms can also be a reflex, but they often have a conscious, brain-directed ingredient as well. Nobody yet has figured how to design a study of the relationship of the brain and orgasm that would pass scientific muster and give us a genuinely useful answer to the question of exactly what brain areas are involved.

MALE BLADDER FUNCTION

Jim noticed increasing changes in his bladder habits as he got older. In his 50s, he would have to get up every so often to go to the bathroom during the night, usually after drinking alcohol. In his 60s, this trip became a nightly occurrence. Now, in his 70s, nature calls two or three times each night. During the day, he sometimes has an almost uncontrollable urge to urinate and must get to the bathroom very quickly. One thing that makes this worse is coffee; he now postpones the first cup until he has arrived at his office. At times now, he experiences a mortifying situation: he will wet his pants a little bit and has to rush to his office and sit down before anyone notices it.

Like our sexual province, our bladder might seem far removed geographically from the brain. However, your brain controls this territory, too, at least in part; most of the time, you decide when it will be in action. When you can't, that's abnormal. Besides their brain connection, these body functions have another thing in common: People don't talk about them, and that includes physicians. The result is that amazingly little is known about some very common changes and complaints.

Getting Up to Urinate at Night

If you're like most men reaching middle age, you're starting to see more of your bathroom at night, probably enough to start thinking your wife is right about remodeling it. Well, go ahead and fix up; you'll be stopping by even more in the next few years. Nine out of 10 men over the age of 60 years will have some change in their urinary habits. Usually, these changes are mild, more annoying than disabling. Most common is getting up at night to urinate. Other common problems are greater urgency when the bladder is full, not being able to start urinating when you want to, and a tendency to dribble after urination seems to be over. All of these, alone or in combination, can make urination a bit of an adventure for an older man. One reason is that older men urinate about the same volume at night as during the day, while younger men do much more of their urinating during the day, and therefore have less water to get rid of at night. The reason for this difference is the action of a hormone, called ADH, that reduces the amount of water flowing out of the kidney. Younger men have higher levels of ADH at night than during the day. In contrast, older men do not have a similar increase in ADH at night, which allows more water to flow from the kidney. More urine accumulates in the bladder, which gets full and signals the brain it is time to get up. In their 50s and 60s, men may need to urinate once or twice a night; in their 70s and 80s, they get up three or four times a night.

The other major problem men find as they get older is that their bladder does not empty properly. As a result, it takes less urine to fill it again. The most common cause of incomplete emptying is enlargement of the prostate gland. The enlarging prostate presses on the tube that leads out of the bladder and interferes with emptying. The bladder may also "overflow," leaking urine in small amounts. Several medications on the market, such as Flo-Max, treat prostate enlargement and alleviate these problems.

Increased Urge to Urinate

As men get older, when their bladder gets full, the urge to urinate comes on more quickly and strongly than when they were younger, and the urge becomes more pressing with advancing years. Certain drinks—coffee or alcohol, for example—and certain medicines, such as diuretics, can make this problem even worse. Coffee causes you to make more urine and stimulates your bladder to empty. That's why, after two cups of coffee in the morning and a long car ride, your first stop is the john. Many people with heart problems take diuretics to get rid of excess water. With these aboard, a person will have repeated episodes of urinary urgency throughout the day or night.

It is also true that the muscles get weaker, particularly the detruser muscle, a crucial muscle required for emptying the bladder. They also become overactive and are more likely to contract, producing the urge to urinate. Several medications can now treat the overactivity of these muscles and reduce the feeling of urgency.

Difficulty Starting to Urinate

Older men may find themselves with a full bladder, rushing to the bathroom only to find that they cannot start urinating. What is happening is that the bladder, as it gets full, gets more and more stretched—just like when you blow up a balloon. Overstretched muscles become weaker, making proper functioning of the bladder difficult. Sometimes a very simple maneuver can help: Press your hands low on your abdomen to increase the pressure on the bladder; this may be all it takes to get urination started. You can ward off problems with starting to urinate by responding to the urge to void as soon as possible, and not letting your bladder get overfull.

Dribbling at the End of Urination

A physician colleague quite succinctly posed this problem as a question: "Still able to wear tan pants?" Dribbling, too, is partly thanks to weakness of the detruser muscle, flubbing its task of forcing urine out of the bladder. Consequently, the force of the urinary stream decreases as your bladder gets emptier. In other words, it is going to take longer to finish urinating than you might expect. Giving your weak detruser muscle the time it needs can be distressing when you need to finish quickly, but most such times you're anxious to accommodate someone else. Our solution? Let 'em wait.

FEMALE BLADDER FUNCTION

Women have many of the same complaints of bladder function as men, including getting up at night to void and having an increased urge to urinate. The treatments for these problems apply equally to women and men.

Leaking Urine

In addition, women often have a problem with leaking of urine when they sneeze, laugh, or cough. Sometimes called stress incontinence, leaking can happen whenever something suddenly increases the pressure within the abdomen. Women who have had children are more likely to experience this problem, which increases markedly as women get older. By the time women are over age 70, the problem affects an estimated one in three. That figure is undoubtedly too low, because many women never discuss this problem with anyone, including their physicians, and are unaware that they may be able to get effective therapy. Many women simply wear pads to absorb the leaking urine. Yet a variety of treatments can help, ranging from exercises to strengthen the muscles that close off the bladder to surgery to tighten up the openings from the bladder. Women also get medications to help keep the bladder from emptying. At one time, estrogen replacement seemed a prospect to help this condition, but recent studies have shown otherwise. Careful urological evaluation and the proper treatment can relieve this problem for many women.

The Brain and Bladder Function

Your bladder is like a reservoir behind a dam. It has two jobs: to store water (or urine) and to periodically let it out. The streams that fill the reservoir are the tubes, called ureters, that go from your kidneys, the source of the water. Like a reservoir, your bladder spends most of its time in storage mode. For example if you urinate 5 or 6 times each day and it takes 2 or 3 minutes to do so, you spend only 10 or 20 minutes actually urinating. But, obviously, your ability to control when and where you urinate is crucial. (An important note: Many problems that affect urination involve kidney trouble or obstruction of the outflow from the bladder. They are outside the interaction between brain and body, and, although we aren't discussing them here, they may need medical attention.)

Your brain is the command center for urination; the bladder operates both automatically and under conscious control. Basically, your bladder is a sack made of muscles that gradually stretch as it fills and expands. The stretched muscles send signals via specific nerves to the spinal cord, which in turn, sends signals back through another set of nerves, telling the bladder to empty. In a newborn, urinating takes place at this reflex level. However, after a child is toilet trained and throughout life, higher centers in the brain take charge and inhibit these reflex mechanisms to make a conscious process. You decide to urinate and these higher centers release the reflex responses of the spinal cord to act. But some injuries to the nervous system can damage these higher centers, removing inhibition and leading to incontinence.

Brain Diseases and the Bladder

The good news about bladder control at middle age and beyond is that someone who treats or makes allowances for the minor complaints will most likely have a well functioning bladder throughout life. But some disorders of the brain and nerves that strike people in their later years can damage the conscious control of urination. The most common of these are stroke and dementia. With illnesses that come on suddenly, such as a stroke or head injury, problems with the bladder often get better gradually. Strokes usually cause damage on only one side of the brain and consequently affect only one side of the body, resulting in incontinence for a week or two. After that—and this is one of the wonders of the brain—the pathway from the brain's undamaged side takes over, bringing bladder functions back toward normal. During the time that bladder control is a problem, the doctor will often order a catheter. In men, an alternative may be some form of external device attached around the penis. A counterpart device may one day be available for women, but none has been invented yet.

People who develop dementias, such as Alzheimer's disease and frontotemporal dementia, have increasing difficulty controlling bladder and bowel function as the disease progresses. A person caring for a friend or relative with mild-to-moderate dementia will find it effective to remind him or her to urinate at specific times during the day. But when the disease is severe, such intervention is very time consuming and often ineffective. At that point, both patient and caregiver are better off if the patient wears pads. Remember, too: people with dementia have the same changes in the bladder muscles as other elderly people, and some of the medications that help with more ordinary complaints can help here, too.

Some illnesses affect bladder function because they alter the nerves that supply the bladder. These illnesses include diabetes, surgical damage to the nerves controlling the bladder (as can occur, for example, in operations on the prostate or bowel), multiple sclerosis, and injury to the spinal cord.

Diabetes can damage the nerves that go to and from the bladder, just as it can the nerves supplying the feet. The nerves coming from the bladder signal when it is full, those going to it signal the muscles to empty the bladder and the outflow valves to open. In extreme situations, the signals that indicate that the bladder is filling up can become increasingly weaker, with the result that the bladder becomes greatly overstretched and never completely empties. Such a pool of urine in the bladder is a set-up for an infection. A similar situation sometimes occurs after major prostate or lower bowel surgery.

When the bladder does not empty normally, several things can be done. One is to use a catheter (a tube that goes directly into the bladder) at least twice a day to empty the bladder. It's true: Many people can learn to put in a catheter themselves; anyone who has the dexterity to write, for example, should be able to do it. However, someone with decreased vision, tremor, or other problems using the hands may not be able to. Then somebody, such as the person's mate, will need to help.

FUTURE TREATMENTS FOR BODILY FUNCTION

Viagra is just the first of a number of drugs that will specifically improve sexual function in men and women. This has become a very hot area of research for pharmaceutical companies.

The more mundane problems with urination are so common that you might consider them a normal part of aging. They don't have to be. As research brings us closer to understanding how these changes work, new treatments are getting more specific. Some of these improvements will come about because we will be better able to treat brain diseases than we are now. For example, for damage to nerves to and from the bladder by diabetes, researchers are evaluating several experimental drugs to see if they can return these damaged nerves to normal function.

WHAT YOU CAN DO ABOUT PROBLEMS WITH BODY FUNCTIONS: DON'T GET UPTIGHT

Most bodily functions are manageable. Sexual function in particular is the good news story of our time: The major change that needs to take place is in an older person's perception of what is normal and what is not. When nearly half of men over 75 had a problem with impotence, many accepted it as normal. There is no need to do so. Most of the time this problem is related to diseases or medications that are common in older people. In addition, Viagra has been an effective form of treatment for erectile dysfunction in men and can also help with the decreased sexual drive brought about by antidepressant medication. Anecdotal evidence suggests that Viagra can also help women with decreased sexual responsiveness, even when due to medications or surgery, such as hysterectomy. However, at this writing studies have just begun and no results for women are available yet.

Urinary problems usually just need to be taken in stride. Most men past their 60s notice that they get up a few times during the night to urinate and that they sometimes take a while to "get things going." Several medications are available to treat urinary urgency and other difficulties.

CHAPTER 9

PROTECTING YOUR SENSES

Guy's father, Charles, lived until he was almost 90. A pediatrician before his retirement, he stayed mentally sharp right up to the end. However, aging is rarely perfect, and, by the time Charles was in his 70s, he had started learning to cope with two limitations: troubles with seeing and hearing.

Charles' vision developed one problem that today is rarely disabling and, later, another that still markedly impairs the quality of life for the elderly. He developed cataracts that required surgery when he was about 70. This was before the lens implant came on the scene, and the surgeries had been only partly successful. Later, in his 80s, he developed degeneration of the nerve cells in his retina, one of the most important parts of the eye for vision. Both his father and brother had also had retinal degeneration. It left him able to read, but only very slowly, using a large magnifying glass. He loved reading, and this tortured pace was a big frustration.

When he conversed with people individually, he could hear them quite well, if they spoke a little more loudly and slowly. However, in a group conversation, such as when the family gathered around a table at Thanksgiving, he was totally handicapped. The background noise was too high, and he had to strain to hear the person next to him. At these times, Charles would become uncharacteristically silent and withdrawn.

We've emphasized how much preserving your mental ability depends upon continued mental and physical activity and a sense of control over your life. The threat of social isolation and physical limitation that can come with diminished sight or hearing can be a major challenge to your feelings of mental vigor and personal capability. Fortunately, if you are like most people whose vision or hearing is disposed to give out, you should be well into your seventh decade or beyond before any loss becomes severe. In that case, your good midlife health habits and your ability to pick up on signs of trouble will help you, when, if ever, you find yourself coping with problems like Charles developed.

Your eyes and ears are two of your hardest-working communicators to your brain. They allow you to receive and interpret information from the world around you and interact with it constantly. Changes in vision and hearing are extremely common with age, which makes it particularly important to try to keep them working as well as possible. Language is the other major link to the outside world for most people. Knowing which changes are normal and which are not, as much as for vision and hearing, is vital for successful aging.

VISION AND AGE

The chances are pretty good that you're reading these words through a pair of glasses; by the time most of us get into our 40s, we are using spectacles, at least to read, if not all the time. Parking reading glasses on your nose may be the best known and most ruefully acknowledged change near midlife, but your vision changes in several subtle ways. The most common shifts take place in how you respond to light and to color, how well you see an object at a distance, and how well you can see fine details of an object. Expect each of these to undergo some alteration in coming years. In later years, usually well into your 70s, you should not be surprised if you develop cataracts. They are quite common and treatment is one of the great advances of medicine in our time.

How Your Eye Works

A camera is a lot like your eye. The light enters at the front of the camera through an opening (the aperture) and then passes through a lens that focuses the light on the film at the back of the camera. In the film, chemicals react to the specific wavelengths of light to store the image. In the front of your eye is an opening (the pupil) and a lens that focuses the light on the back of the eye. Like the film in a camera, a sheet of nerve cells (called the retina) at the back of your eye responds to the wavelengths of light. Fortunately, the parallel of the living retina and chemical film falls apart here: Unlike when you're using a camera, you don't have to pop out the film and process it to bring out the image. The retina's nerve cells send signals over specific pathways to the brain areas that form images. Then, other parts of the brain interpret the image in terms of your previous experience, memories, and emotions.

Changes in Response to Light

Glare sensitivity is a common complaint, starting as early as age 50. If you find you like driving at night less than you once did, this sensitivity is probably the reason. For a few moments after passing the bright lights of an approaching car, you have difficulty making out the details of the road. This sensitivity to glare involves all parts of your eye: The pupil is slower to constrict, the lens gradually transmits light less well, and the nerves in the retina work differently. Some cases of glare sensitivity are due to early cataracts and may be helped by cataract surgery.

Changes in Visual Acuity

Visual acuity is the measurement of how well you see small or distant objects. Your eye doctor tests it by having you look at an eye chart. Visual acuity changes quite slowly with age. For example, if you still have 20/20 vision at age 50, you might drop to 20/40 by the time you are 90. To put it another way, at 90, you may have to be twice as close to an object as you were at 50, in order to see it clearly. This type of change, which is considered normal, is reflected in how well you can read or recognize people or signs. The usual progression is from no glasses, to reading glasses, to bifocals or trifocals; and for some, to large-print books or newspapers.

Mostly, these changes are due to the difficulty your lens has in changing shape, which it must do when you shift from looking at up-close objects to those at a distance. We call this lens adjustment "accommodation," and it is like changing the focal point of a camera. Because it normally declines with age, by the time you are 50, you may have to hold objects farther away while you read. When your arms are not long enough anymore, you'll have to get bifocal glasses or contact lenses to correct the problem.

Cataracts

It is said that the impressionist painter, Claude Monet, lost his use of blues and greens for a period of time, when he was older. As it turned out, this was because he was developing cataracts. The lens at the front of his eye thickened and gained a yellow tint, like old bottle glass. Less and less light got through to the retina and the short (blue) wave-lengths were filtered out. When Monet had cataract surgery, even the cataract surgery of 100 years ago, he regained his color perception of blues and greens.

The development of cataracts is, in fact, so common that it is almost considered a normal part of aging. About one-half of people between 75 and 85 will have significant loss of vision from cataracts. The cause is not clear, but prolonged exposure to ultraviolet light is a predisposing factor. Those working in bright sunlight, like fishermen or policemen, should use dark glasses that protect the eyes from these ultraviolet (short-wave) rays. Not all sunglasses do this, and plastic lenses are much better than glass lenses.

CATARACT SURGERY

We cannot think of a procedure that has been more successful in improving the lives of so many older people than the new cataract surgery developed during the last 20 years. In the old days, the lens was removed in a surgery that required a week in the hospital. The patient, like Guy's father, then wore either special contact lenses or very thick glasses the rest of his life. Today in cataract surgery, the lens with the cataract is replaced by a lens implant. It is an outpatient procedure and takes about 20 minutes. It leaves you with near normal vision with regular glasses.

If you get cataracts in both eyes, your eye surgeon will usually fix only one at a time. In very rare instances, the operated eye can develop an infection, which can be damaging. Fortunately, if infection does occur, it usually responds to antibiotics. This new form of cataract surgery has caught on very quickly and is still being improved. Even though it is a specialized field of ophthalmology, most communities have at least one well-trained cataract surgeon.

Retinal Degeneration

The second most common reason why an older person has trouble with vision is difficulty with the back part of the eye (the retina), the equivalent of the film in a camera. This problem, called retinal degeneration, usually progresses slowly with age.

In Charles' case, the process started when he was about 80. He began having trouble seeing the small print in newspapers and books. For several years, he was able to read normal print using a magnifying glass. Toward the end of his life, he had to use large-print books and newspapers. All told, he had this problem for over 10 years but was still able to read independently at age 90.

Retinal degeneration is also called macular degeneration. The major problem develops in the center of the retina, called the macula, which is the area involved in seeing small objects, such as letters. A person is not blind; for example, he or she can still see objects in a room and people.

The disorder typically makes its appearance when individuals are in their 60s and 70s and can progress slowly over a decade or more. Typically, this problem runs in families, and researchers have already identified specific genes linked to it. This is good news for our chances to someday work out how to stop it before it starts. However, it can also develop without a family history; some research suggests that as many as a third of the over-75 population may have it to some degree. We also know that cigarette smoking, and possibly excess exposure to sunlight, may have something to do with the development of this disorder.

Retinal degeneration begins with the development of new, tiny blood vessels under the retina. These abnormal blood vessels can suddenly break, causing bleeding and a sudden decrease in vision. One of the new advances, using laser surgery, can now prevent and treat this problem by sealing the small vessels shut. Another, even newer form of treatment called photodynamic therapy destroys the new blood vessels, protecting the eye from damage.

High dose of a combination of dietary supplements—zinc, the antioxidants vitamin C and vitamin E, and beta-carotene—slow the progression of the disease but do not prevent it from appearing. Using one of these supplements alone was not as effective as the combination. This finding, based on following over 4,500 individuals for over 6 years, strongly suggests that this process can be slowed down. How long the benefit lasts is not yet known.

HEARING AND AGE

Changes in hearing are so common in midlife that the line between normal and abnormal is quite blurred, as with changes in seeing. If your hearing starts to decline, it will most likely be in the form of increasing difficulty understanding what people are saying, especially in a noisy room or when several people are talking at once. This can happen to you quite early—when you are in your 50s is not unusual—and your chances of getting some hearing loss, perhaps a significant loss, grow as you get older. The first effect you may notice is difficulty hearing sounds at high frequencies, but, gradually, sounds of lower frequencies seem harder to hear, too. Men are more likely than women to have hearing loss, perhaps because men may be exposed to more loud noises, as, for example, in noisy work environments or using guns.

High-Tone Hearing Loss

Sound travels through the air in waves at different frequencies, that is, a certain number of sound waves per second. Lower sounds send fewer waves, higher sounds, more. In your inner ear, a part designed like a xylophone, the cochlea, receives sound. Tiny hairs are the equivalent of each key of the xylophone. Specific sets of hairs start to vibrate when a sound of a particular frequency hits them. The hairs are connected to nerves that send the sound signals to the brain, which then recognizes the individual sounds. As we age, some hairs in the xylophone-like apparatus have more trouble functioning. These are the hairs that catch higher pitched sounds and are also the likeliest to be damaged by loud noises.

Quite a few studies are trying to measure whether our increasingly noisy environment is contributing to more hearing loss with aging. You may have noticed airport workers and construction workers now wear protectors over their ears to avoid this problem. And many of us have wondered if former President Clinton earned his two hearing aids from exposure to loud music in the 1960s and 1970s.

The result of high-tone hearing loss is that you become less able to understand speech, particularly when the background noise is loud. You may be able to identify individual words, but find it hard to catch the whole sentence. Everybody with this kind of hearing loss uses word clues, does a lot of guessing, and attempts to read lips to compensate.

Being unable to understand sentences may not be wholly the fault of those tiny hairs. At midlife, we slow down in how fast our brains process the information coming in from all our senses. That's why, in predicting how well a person will respond to a hearing aid, one of the technical measurements looks for the relationship between your ability to identify words and identify sentences. If you can recognize words and sentences about equally, the tiny hairs will be considered the culprit, and your ear doctor would expect you to do well with a hearing aid. If you can understand individual words, but not sentences, the sound signals may be moving too slowly along the nerve circuits after the inner ear. We call this a central hearing problem and a hearing aid may not help.

Hearing Aids—The First Line of Defense

The hearing aid is the first line of defense against problems with hearing. And fortunately they have become much easier to use and much less obtrusive. They have become smaller, more reliable, and more adjustable to individual problems. There are a number of reasons why people are reluctant to use hearing aids. Probably the first is pure vanity—the idea that use of a hearing aid is a sign of aging. Others may have tried older models, found them hard to use, and given up. And, undeniably, there is cost—they are not cheap.

We think that having a small, barely visible device in your ear is highly preferable to having people think you're out of it because you only hear half of what they are saying. If you have tried older models and been discouraged, try again, because progress in this area has been remarkable. It is true they are not cheap but they are covered by Medicare and most forms of insurance, specifically because hearing properly is recognized as such an essential part of living independently.

One situation we know is not vanity and is certainly understandable: Some people have trouble making the adjustments on a hearing aid, particularly if they have poor use of their fingers or poor vision. In that case, rather than letting the person opt out, someone else can easily adjust the hearing aid for them.

Assisted Listening Devices

Assisted listening devices, sometimes called ALDs, are a great advance in the amplification of sound. ALDs run the gamut from devices to amplify your telephone and TV, to systems wired to boost conversations in a room. The basic idea is the same for all these devices: Place a microphone near the source of the sound to send the sound signal to a modified hearing aid. The merit here is that the listener gets a much better signal-to-noise ratio, that is, you hear more of the sounds you want and much less of the background noise. Assisted listening devices can be particularly helpful for someone with a progressive hearing loss who is losing the benefit of a hearing aid.

Cochlear Implants for Hearing Loss

In some people, there is severe hearing loss because the xylophone-like structure of tiny hairs no longer responds. This is true of children with some forms of congenital deafness or deafness from some infections. In adults, there can be a progressive failure for the same reason.

For someone with this type of severe hearing loss, cochlear implants are a possibility. A cochlear implant is a listening device placed just past the inner ear; it delivers sound by small wires directly to the nerve cells designed to respond to sounds. It is a surgical procedure and only people with severely limited ability to recognize single words—in other words, whose hearing loss approaches deafness—are candidates for it. For three out of four people with this type of hearing problem, the cochlear implant can improve hearing. Age does not rule out a cochlear implant, but having been severely deaf a long time does. The longer significant hearing loss has gone on, the less likely an implant will work. The technology for implants is still evolving, and this promising approach to hearing loss may come into wider use in the future. One impediment is the cost, which can be as high as $40,000 for the implant and its surgical placement. Fortunately, most insurance plans will cover this cost.

Other Ways to Assist Hearing

Even when neither a hearing aid nor an assisted listening device is the answer, there are other remedies. Everyone will communicate best when they avoid difficult listening conditions. The idea is to speak distinctly and hold down the background noise, such as from a TV set or lots of people talking all at once. For TV watching or telephone conversation, you can even obtain nonwearable aids, such as chair-side amplifiers. The point is, communication is extremely important and everybody gains by trying everything to make it as successful as possible.

Marilyn has an 87-year-old relative who is an example of how good imagination can help maintain communication with others, even with a considerable hearing loss. Her hearing problems started when she was in her 60s. She first noticed it when people were gathered around the dining room table and many people were talking at once. She could hear and understand the person next to her, but could not understand what others were saying. She ignored these problems for several years, until her children commented that she kept asking them to repeat things. She hadn't realized she was doing that. She had her hearing examined and discovered that she had a decreased ability to hear words and sentences. The doctor thought she had a mixture of both an inner ear and central hearing problem. She used hearing aids successfully for about 10 years, but then her understanding of what people were saying got worse. She began to use an assisted listening device and still does. In a noisy restaurant, she holds the microphone close to the mouth of the person who is speaking to her and usually can understand. But she can no longer make out conversation over the telephone. Her children got the idea that she would be able to remain in touch with them by using a fax machine and, more recently e-mail. That was a stroke of genius: Every week, she writes letters about what she is doing and sends them to close family members. These letters have become such a pleasure to everyone that she is now in much more regular contact with her family than she was years ago.

How Do Sensory Systems Work?

Even though our sensory systems—vision, hearing, smell, taste, and touch—are obviously different from each other, the brain has them organized in a similar way. The specialized parts of the body—eyes, ears, nose, mouth, and skin—receive messages from the outside and transmit them to the part of the brain that is specialized for that particular source of information.

All the sensory systems have a peripheral (outside the brain) and central (brain) component. The peripheral component detects signals in the environment and sends them to the brain. In seeing and hearing, the signals are in wave form, light waves or sound waves, and the eye and ear nerve cells are specialized to pick up the waves and convert them into messages the brain can use. In the retina, nerve cells respond to specific wave-lengths of light to recognize colors, and in the ear, specific nerve cells respond to sounds at a particular frequency. With so much exposure, these peripheral nerve cells are the most vulnerable part of each of the sensory systems.

Your brain has separate areas for vision and hearing. Each peripheral source uses its own pathway of nerves to get into the brain and its own specific parts of the brain handle that sensory information. Eventually, the brain has to put these independent incoming signals together as meaningful information. For example, when you look at an object, your eyes send your brain an image of four legs, a seat, and a back. Then a particular area of your brain puts these components together as the recognizable object, a chair. Similarly, areas in your brain recognize a specific set of eyes, ears, nose, and mouth as a person's face, a set of letters as a word, or a series of sounds as a tune. To do this, these processing centers take information from around your brain, process it into a recognizable form, such as a word or picture, and then compare it with what you already know. If the object is something you ordinarily use or see, such as a pencil or TV screen, this adding-up goes very rapidly. If an object is unfamiliar or complex, for example, a word in a foreign language or a street sign, it takes longer to put the information together to make it meaningful.

As we age, the speed of putting the component pieces of information into a meaningful whole seems to get slightly slower. Therefore, some mental tasks that used to operate very quickly, such as recognizing someone's face, take longer than they used to.

LANGUAGE AND AGE

Language is our link to the outside world. It is so effortless that most of the time that we take it for granted. Fortunately, ability to use language changes little with age. In fact, some aspects of language ability, such as the richness of vocabulary, actually improve.

For language to function normally, our ability to both take in and put out language must work well. The intake side of language depends on our being able to hear what someone is saying, or read what someone has written, and then to understand it. The output side of language is our production of coherent speech.

Language has top priority in life from the moment we utter our first cry. If you doubt it, consider the fact that language and walking develop at about the same age in almost every child who is normal. Not only that, but regardless of the language a child is born into (including sign language), the stages of becoming able to speak—from babbling, to single words, to phrases, and then sentences—appear at about the same time in all children. And in all cases, our ability as babies to understand language comes before our ability to express words. The major influence from the environment is to instill the particular language or languages we will speak. Our inborn brain mechanisms for learning language reside in areas of the brain that two nineteenth-century physicians first found, and we use these areas to acquire language until we are 10 or 12 years old. After that, to learn a new language, we use different brain mechanisms. The parts of the brain we use when we learn a language later in life include not only the original language systems, but other parts as well. It is as if we no longer process language as a special function, but now use the same brain mechanisms to learn it that we use for learning many other things. That explains why a child younger than age 10 learns a new language so much more quickly and completely than an adult. The child is still using the brain areas dedicated to acquiring early language—specific mechanisms we don't tap into when we are older.

Understanding Language

Unless you have problems with vision or hearing, your grasp of language will be remarkably stable across your life span and preserved as you grow older. Your understanding for the words or types of sentences you need in reading a magazine or newspaper or listening to the news will not change, and your vocabulary may even improve with age.

But the speed of the information coming to you will begin to make a difference when you start getting into your 60s. When information, particularly spoken, is presented rapidly, older people understand it less well than younger ones. The decrease in your ability to process quickly presented oral information will affect how well you comprehend information from, for example, a news broadcast. You might even find you enjoy reading more: Since you read at your own speed and can go back over what you read, speed has less influence on your understanding of written material. You'll also find you look forward more to seeing your Southern friends; they speak slower.

One advantage of the computer is that it depends on the written word. Given the fact that vocabulary and reading ability do not decline and may even improve with age, it's not surprising that the fastest-growing group of new computer users in the United States is over the age of 65.

Storytelling

Around the world, and even in America, but perhaps with less recognition, the older population is responsible for passing along the wisdom of previous generations. In fact, many aspects of the output side of language—speaking—go on working very well as people get older, and storytelling is one of them. In studies with people listening to older and younger storytellers, the older ones are rated as being more skilled than the younger ones, and older storytellers often include more vivid details than people who are younger. Older people tend to express themselves differently than younger people. They tend to use more words to get across an idea or to convey information, both in writing and in speaking. It's possible that older people use more words to convey an idea because the process of selecting words slows down slightly with age. If this slowness leads to difficulty recalling exactly the word one wants to use, the result may be to use multiple related words when, in fact, a single one could have been used. And that may be what enriches the older storyteller's tales.

Problems with Naming

If there is one area of language that bothers everybody as they get into midlife, it is a problem with naming—those so-called "senior moments" we discussed in chapter 1, "Maintaining Your Memory." No question, coming up with the name of a person or even the name of an object becomes gradually more difficult as people get older.

It is worth emphasizing that the problem you might have coming up with a name doesn't mean that, for some reason, you no longer know it. You know the name; you're just having trouble recalling it. We usually can come up with loads of information about someone we can't name—when we first met them, what they do, their dog's name, even what they look like—just not their name. Often a simple cue, such as the first letter of someone's name, is all it takes to bring it back. In other words, the information is all there; you just have trouble bringing it to mind. Very often, a few minutes or hours later, the name will suddenly pop up. Many researchers study this problem of recalling names, but they haven't determined exactly why it gets worse as we age. One possibility is that, as part of the general slowing in language processing we've described, it takes longer for your brain to collect the multiple bits of information that identify the correct name.

One of the most important ways of safeguarding your dexterity with language is to follow a health regimen that will reduce your risk of stroke (see page 264).

RESEARCH IN THE SENSES

It may sound like science fiction, but for people who have impaired vision due to retinal degeneration, researchers are developing methods to bypass the retina entirely. That is, they are studying techniques to electronically send images from the outside world to the brain areas that receive visual information. This technology uses a screen to detect objects and then sends the images to electrodes placed on the areas of the brain that receive visual information. Technology like this is actually being used experimentally—individuals with acquired blindness can detect light and dark shapes, but not the fine details necessary to recognize faces or words. But that will surely come.

Similarly, in a new experimental treatment that may ultimately be preferable to cochlear implants for acquired deafness, researchers are bypassing the peripheral hearing mechanisms and sending signals to the parts of the brain that detect and discriminate sounds. This too has developed enough for people to test it.

WHAT YOU CAN DO ABOUT PROTECTING YOUR SENSES

Communicating—that is, being able to hear what people say, read, and express yourself—are essential to productive aging. The most common reasons for deafness can be helped by hearing aids—use them. Similarly, a common cause of decreased vision, cataracts, can be cured by surgery.

Other causes of decreasing vision are like other diseases in which nerve cells die; we are learning the genetics and mechanisms, but don't yet have treatments. However, there is evidence that lifestyle factors influence macular degeneration, particularly smoking and exposure to sunlight. This is a good reason to quit smoking and an excellent argument for sunglasses.

CHAPTER 10

HOW TO KEEP YOUR BALANCE— LITERALLY

The audience became silent as the conductor, Yehudi Menuhin, came through the side door and made his way through the orchestra to the podium. He lifted his baton and began to conduct a concert that spanned two hours, with only a brief intermission. The audience rose to its feet to acknowledge another outstanding performance. No surprise in one sense, because this conductor had been giving performances of this sort for over 50 years. Then again, the man was now 80 years old!

Conducting requires not only the understanding of music but also great physical energy and stamina. We say to ourselves, "How exceptional," but it's not. The pianist Arthur Rubinstein played into his 90s, as did the cellist Pablo Casals. Many other musical performers and conductors also performed at a high level until a well advanced age. In a different kind of virtuosity, at least one gentleman we know continued to run the Boston Marathon until he was in his 80s. Older people can continue to function physically very well, particularly if they have been performing at a physically high level throughout their lives. This doesn't mean you suddenly have to start training for the Olympics. It means you simply have to get up and move.

There are changes in how you perform physical activities as you age—changes in strength, flexibility, posture, and balance. But there are things you can do to minimize these changes and we will discuss them. Improving your movements, particularly balance, is important to avoid falls. The prevention of falls is one of the most important things you can do to avoid unnecessary disability. In addition to improving your balance, you can also make changes to your home to help make it more fall-proof.

FACING UP TO SLOWING DOWN

No matter how much you practice or exercise, the truth is you simply won't be able to perform many physical activities as well as 20-somethings can. For example, most older people can no longer hit a golf ball as far, or run for a ball in tennis as quickly. If these abilities didn't change, there would be no need for a senior golf tour (for those over 50) or a senior tennis circuit (for those over 35, no less!). Changes in our ability to move also affect such simple everyday activities as walking, getting in and out of chairs, and climbing stairs. Exercise can lessen these changes but it cannot prevent them.

Many things account for changes in mobility. As we age, our joints may be stiffer and our muscles somewhat weaker. Our reflexes are slower and our balance is not as good. These changes occur in people who are clinically healthy and therefore we consider them "normal" aspects of aging. But "normal" is still a relative term. Much can be done to minimize these changes.

Muscle Strength

Muscles get weaker as we get older, a phenomenon accentuated for people living sedentary lives. An afternoon spent playing bridge, watching television, or reading a book may be enjoyable and rewarding in its own way, but these activities do nothing for your muscle tone, strength, or endurance. It does not take much exercise to make a difference, though. Just walking two to three times each week can help, as can exercise classes and low-impact aerobics. These activities will keep your muscle strength up to the level it should be.

Joint Stiffness

Stiffness and limitation of movement of joints can be part of the problem. Joints are designed to move. When a joint is restricted in its movement, it gets even stiffer. One of the major benefits of physical therapy programs is to get joints moving and to recover mobility.

Changes in Posture

For us to move correctly, information coming into the brain has to be put together and used. As we get older, parts of the brain systems needed to integrate incoming sensory information in order to make movements may not function as well. This is probably why some older people tend to shuffle when they walk, have difficulty turning quickly, and have changes in posture, marked by a tendency to slump over. These integrating systems also respond to exercises that concentrate on movement and balance.

Changes in Balance

Balance is the most complicated part of movement because it calls for the brain to integrate three different functions: vision, sensory input, and information about balance from your inner ears. Simple exercises, such as standing on one leg or standing with one foot in front of the other, can improve balance. Balance will respond to this kind of training just as it does during athletic training in a younger person, if not to the same degree. One reason it is particularly important to work on maintaining balance is the prevention of falls. Studies indicate that the lack of balance is the best predictor of who will have a fall.

How Your Brain Controls Movement and Balance

When you reach for an object, walk downstairs, or roll over in bed, your brain must coordinate a series of commands to nerves and muscles and interpret feedback from your joints and other signals of your body's position.

Some movements, such as standing, sitting, or walking are virtually automatic. We don't think about them except to start the action, say, deciding to stand up. Then basic reflex mechanisms in the brain take over the movement. In contrast are movements you learn and must think about each step of the way, as when you first learn to write. With practice, however, learned movements also become virtually automatic. For example, a guitar player playing the rapid part of a song cannot be thinking about each finger movement. He or she has learned a complex motor program by repeatedly practicing, first playing the piece very slowly, and then more rapidly. Your ability to recall and use these motor programs does not decline with age, as long as you keep them intact by practicing.

Sometimes even automatic movements, such as walking, may have to be relearned. After injury or replacement of a hip or knee a person has to consciously think about putting weight on the affected limb and then, very cautiously, how to move it. Gradually, with practice, walking again becomes a natural movement.

Learning a new motor movement involves specific areas in the brain. These areas feed their information to nerve cells in the motor cortex, the area in the brain involved with the initiation of movement. Signals from the motor cortex nerve cells travel downstream, through the spinal cord, just as messages are sent through a telephone cable. At intervals are nerves that leave the spinal cord. They carry signals to specific muscles. The muscles provide the strength that makes the movement possible.

To move properly, you also need sensory feedback telling your brain, for example, where your feet are and how they are moving, or the position of your hand as you reach for a cup of coffee. The sensory signals arise from special nerve endings in the skin, responding to pressure and the feeling of movement and, in joints, relaying changes in position. These signals return through nerves to the spinal cord and then back up to the brain. Specific parts of the brain, such as the cerebellum, integrate this incoming information and use it to modify movements. You can use this sensory information to make certain movements with eyes closed, or when you pick up the telephone next to your bed in the dark.

Balancing involves these sensory systems plus two others: your vision, and the specific balancing mechanisms in your inner ears. Vision tells you where you are in space, whether you are standing still or moving, and in what direction. Similarly, the balancing mechanisms inside your ears signal what position you are in, whether you are moving, and in what direction. One balancing mechanism in your ear is a structure called the otolith which consists of microscopic stones, smaller than a grain of salt, balanced on individual hairs. When you move, these stones move and signal the brain. In older people, some of these stones can fall off and interfere, often quite nastily, with balancing mechanisms.

You can get along quite well using only two of these balancing mechanisms. For example, you can balance nicely in the dark if the sensory feedback from your feet and the balancing mechanisms in your ears is working normally. One reason an older person may have trouble balancing at night when he gets out of bed to use the bathroom is that, in the dark, the sensory information from his legs or ears, or both, may not be good enough to compensate for the lack of visual input.

IT'S NEVER TOO LATE TO TAKE UP PHYSICAL ACTIVITY

One of our colleagues was a very hard working scientist, often involved in experiments that went on for days. In his 60s, he decided to relinquish administrative responsibilities but to continue his research activities. This allowed him time to return to playing tennis, something he had not had time to do for over 40 years. He approached tennis the same way he did his science; carefully analyzing his strengths and weaknesses, and working with a mentor on occasion. Over the intervening 15 years his tennis game has gotten better and better, so much so that he has a new criterion for retirement—the day one of us beats him on the court.

More and more we have become a nation of couch potatoes—more accurately, desk and car potatoes. We sit, behind a desk or behind a wheel, partly by necessity and partly by pure laziness. We sometimes have good intentions and carry with us the unused membership to a health club. Still, more of us are recognizing the importance of regular physical activity in order to be at our best.

Millions of people now hitting middle age have taken up walking, swimming, aerobics and dance classes, and even "pumping iron," reaping the benefits of physical activity at multiple levels. The same is true for those much older. Exercise helps improve your flexibility, your balance, and your strength. In addition, it has positive effects on your bone structure and cardiovascular fitness. Moreover, a growing number of studies link physical activity and the maintenance of cognitive performance, that is, the preservation of your thinking and memory abilities. Finally, exercise just makes you feel better about yourself.

It may not make too much difference what you do, so long as you "just do it." This gets you out of the sedentary mindset. Some feel that one reason women live longer than men is that women generally have more of the responsibility for cooking, cleaning, and shopping, all of which involve considerable amounts of walking, bending, standing, and lifting. Regardless of daily habits, most people getting to their middle years need to build regular exercise into their lives and to give it high priority. And illness actually heightens the need, rather than lessening it. Many cardiologists send patients to exercise programs after a heart attack or heart surgery. Likewise, many orthopedists send patients to regular exercise programs after hip or knee problems have developed. When you start a program like this for medical reasons, it can set up a pattern of continuing exercise with benefits for the rest of your life. But why wait until illness strikes? Start now!

We like to ride bicycles and do it as much as possible, but weather and work prevent us from biking as regularly as we would like. We have therefore tried to find exercises that fit easily into a busy schedule. We try to do sit ups, knees bent, each morning and ride a stationary bicycle for 15 to 20 minutes. Inspired by Miriam Nelson, author of *Strong Women Stay Young,* we (Yes, Guy too!) also try to use ankle weights and small dumbbells (5 or 10 pounds) in a few simple exercises a few times a week while sitting and doing other things, such as talking on the telephone or watching television.

FUTURE RESEARCH IN MOVEMENT AND BALANCE

Many in today's older generation have lived very sedentary lives. This is not as true for the age group coming up behind them. Recently, we were at a meeting in Washington, D.C., on a beautiful spring day. During lunchtime so many office workers who appeared to be in their 30s and 40s were out walking and running that the capital looked like one enormous track meet. These walkers' and runners' more active lifestyles will lead to fewer problems with movement and balance as they get older.

Better fitness research is also going on that will give us more specific ideas about designing exercise programs to reduce problems with movement and balance. Studies in this area with respect to the elderly began only about a decade ago, and the results are just beginning to come into the mainstream.

FALLS

It was a beautiful day, warm for January, and we decided to go for a walk. Guy went upstairs and put on some boots with thick, cleated soles. Coming down the stairs, the toe of his right boot caught in the carpet of the stairs and down he went. As he fell, he felt a snap in his knee, and, when he landed, he could not straighten out his leg. He had snapped the tendon that attaches his kneecap to the muscles of his thigh. After surgery and months of physical therapy, his walking gradually returned to normal. Going down stairs is still a bit of a problem. As a matter of fact, he gives every staircase he meets an extra measure of wary respect.

Every year, about one-third of people over the age of 65 report at least one serious fall, and the problem gets worse as individuals get older, especially for women. For a lot of reasons, an older person may fall quite unexpectedly and without any apparent cause. In many cases, however, the cause is clear. A person trips over an extension cord, a rug slides out from under her feet on a slippery floor, or he misses the bottom step on a stair and pitches forward. Even shoes can be a problem, as Guy can attest.

Why People Fall

Let's try an experiment. With someone standing beside you to steady you if you start to fall, put your feet together, one foot right in front of the other. Now lean to one side. What happens? You don't have to lean very far before you have to put your foot out to keep your balance. If you shift your center of gravity by leaning too far, you either have to counterbalance that shift in weight by moving other parts of your body—a shoulder or arm back in the other direction—or you have to move your leg to catch yourself. In other words, you have to make a postural adjustment with your body or your feet. Your ability to adjust your posture tends to decrease with age. Older people are slower in making the movements required to maintain balance, so slight obstacles that would not bother a younger person may topple an elderly person. Further, when elderly people do fall, they are more likely to injure themselves.

How to Prevent Falls

PHYSICAL EXERCISE. The best way to minimize the changes that age brings in balance and strength is regular physical activity. Ask yourself what physical activity you get pleasure from—walking, swimming, yoga, tai chi? If you enjoy it, then you will do it regularly, which is the important thing.

RECOGNIZE THE DANGEROUS TIMES FOR FALLING. The first line of prevention, especially if you are heading into your 70s or so, is to recognize the danger that suddenly standing up from a lying or sitting position can pose. You should get up slowly—not immediately jump up and try to get moving as you did when you were younger. If you have been at rest for a while, it is sometimes helpful if you exercise your feet and legs a little bit before you get up, just to start the blood moving out of your legs and back into circulation. We advise some of our elderly patients to sit on the edge of their bed or chair for a minute or two, flexing their calf muscles and moving their feet around before they get up. We tell them to be sure to have something to hang onto. If they start to fall, they can sit back down and start over again.

When someone has been bedridden for a while, the first days and weeks of getting up again are particularly dangerous. The reflexes involved with standing and balancing—the postural adjusting mechanisms—weren't being used and essentially went to sleep. It takes time, often two to three weeks, for these reflex systems to respond normally.

Risks from Fear of Falling

We have a two-year-old grandson who seems to fall 20 to 30 times a day, each time bouncing back up again. Older people, on the other hand, with the same stumbles, often break bones, particularly hips or arms. In addition, they may develop fear of falling, called fallophobia. Even people who have never actually fallen and hurt themselves can become overly cautious. Getting up out of bed at night to go to the bathroom becomes a major psychological hurdle. This fear is important to recognize, for both the person and the person's family, because fallophobia can lead to increasing social isolation and increasing inactivity. Sometimes offering a supporting arm or hand is all that is required to help a person take the first few steps.

Future Research in Falls

Despite the frequency of falls in older people, only recently have medical researchers studied who is at risk for falls and how to prevent them. The major focus is discovering what types of exercises improve balance and strength. It is likely that the research will lead to specific guidelines about exercises that can minimize falls.

WHAT YOU CAN DO ABOUT FALLS:
MAKE YOUR HOME FALL-PROOF

Most falls occur in the home, in particular trouble spots. Here are some things you can do to minimize the danger.

- *Improve Lighting.* You should be careful going into a room without the lights on. For example, use a night-light to help you see your way from your bed to the bathroom.
- *Watch Out For Rugs and Chairs.* Rugs and chairs can slide when you step or sit on them. Put pads under rugs and cups under chair feet to prevent them from slipping. Remember that bathroom rugs can present the same hazard as rugs on other floors in your home. In one study, the most frequent single cause for falls was tripping over the edge of rugs and carpets. Double-sided rug tape can secure these edges.
- *Put Rails on All Stairs and Use Them.* Going downstairs is a genuine risk at any age. That's why every local building code in the United States now requires handrails. In adolescence and our 20s, we don't have the patience to use them, but, as we get older, failing to isn't very smart. Train yourself to use the handrails at all times. Look at your feet as you go down stairs to be sure you are placing them correctly, and consider putting a stripe of white on the bottom step so you can tell where it is. This may be particularly important on cellar stairs where the lighting may be poor. Install and use handrails on outside steps, which become particularly hazardous with rain or snow.
- *Make Your Bathroom User-Friendly.* Install a higher toilet seat so that the toilet is easier to use. Put in handrails so that you will have something to hold onto as you use the toilet and get in or out of the bathtub or shower. The bars of your towel racks are not strong enough; if you start to fall, these will probably pull out of the wall. You need good, solid supports.

All these technical changes are fine, and important, but what will help most is for you to improve your balance by exercising.

CHAPTER 11

FAINTING, DIZZINESS, AND YOUR BRAIN

FAINTING

Recently, during a prolonged Christmas Eve service, an attractive woman who appeared to be in her 50s suddenly slumped to the floor at the back of the church where she had been standing. Every physician in the congregation sprang to her aid, despite her protestations that she was all right. Going out into the cool air soon revived her, and she quickly recovered.

We see a number of people as patients who complain of feeling light-headed and dizzy. It is not entirely clear what they mean by those commonly used words. In one instance, their blood pressure may be too low; they are not getting enough blood to their brain, and are in danger of fainting. Alternatively, something may be affecting the balancing mechanisms in their ear and making them dizzy. So even though they are using similar words, the mechanisms are quite different.

People who faint almost always do so while standing. Usually a person has a brief warning, a feeling of being lightheaded, dizzy, wobbly, or weak at the knees. If the person sits or lies down quickly enough, the symptoms will pass. If not, the person faints, meaning that he or she slumps to the floor, usually without injury. Once a person has fainted, he or she may recover very quickly. Arms or legs may make a few jerky movements, then they may shake their head and become oriented in a minute or two, often embarrassed by the circumstances and anxious to get up again. Fainting usually leaves no lingering confusion, headache, or other symptoms. Certain environments seem to promote fainting: hot, stuffy rooms; the sight of blood; fear of injury (even a minor "injury" like an injection); or standing immobile for a long time.

Why Do People Faint?

Adults of all ages can faint when the brain does not get enough blood, which can happen for two reasons. Most of the time, the heart is normal, but may beat too slowly because of an emotional response. This is what happened if you were ever about to get an injection and fainted just as the needle approached your arm. Your heart slowed down as a response to this emotional trauma, and not enough blood was pumped up to your brain.

A more likely scenario in fainting is that not enough blood circulates for your heart to pump. This will happen when blood pools in your legs after you have been standing for a long time, as the woman in church had been. When you change position from lying down to standing up, your body has to make adjustments to keep your blood pressure up. Initially, standing constricts the blood vessels to the legs so that blood doesn't pool there. But if you stand still long enough, this constricting mechanism may gradually loosen up and blood will pool in your lower extremities. You will first become light-headed, and then you may faint. More than once, we have seen a striking picture in the newspaper of Queen Elizabeth II reviewing her troops with a supine Grenadier at her feet. Most professional soldiers who must stand at attention for a long time learn how to rock in place and flex their leg muscles to avoid this pooling of blood in their lower extremities.

Some people faint when they stand up after they have been sitting or lying down for a long period of time. Their bodies don't make the necessary internal adjustments when they move from a lying to a standing position. Many medications taken by older people make this problem worse or even cause it, especially those that lower blood pressure. For example, people with Parkinson's disease tend to have low blood pressure, and when they take anti-Parkinson drugs, which tend to lower blood pressure even more, they get light-headed and dizzy on standing. People who become light-headed on standing should carefully review their medications with their physician. Many medications can affect blood pressure adversely, and medicines can be additive in their effects, meaning that you can take one drug without trouble, but if you take it with another medicine, the combination can lower blood pressure significantly.

Men, particularly older men, may faint while urinating. The fainting episode usually occurs at the end of urination when one gets up at night. It is not entirely clear why—perhaps the sudden emptying of the bladder leads to a slowing of the heart. This scenario for fainting may sound funny, but it is not funny when it happens. Bathrooms are dangerous places to fall, with protruding edges and hard surfaces like toilet bowls and sinks. This type of fainting can be avoided by sitting down to urinate.

Fainting for Unusual Reasons

The middle-aged wife of one of our colleagues had stopped to do an errand, returned to her car, and was driving home when suddenly she realized that the car sounded very odd, with a dragging sound from the right front fender. She stopped and saw that the whole right side had been bashed in. She was quite awake, but scared. She called her husband, who came to get her and saw that she had hit a guard rail about 50 yards back from where she stopped. It seemed clear that she had a moment of unconsciousness, without warning and without any aftereffects. We call this atypical fainting, a fainting episode that occurs when sitting, or even lying down. This episode had two possible reasons. The first was some form of brief epileptic seizure. That was ruled out with an electroencephalogram (also called an EEG) that showed her readings were normal. The other possibility was that she had experienced an irregular heartbeat.

To explore this possibility, our friend's wife wore a cardiac monitor for 24 hours, which revealed that she was having short bursts of abnormal heart rhythm, an arrhythmia. She responded to heart medications and is now doing well.

DIZZINESS

The sudden loss of balance or a sudden spinning sensation, which we refer to as dizziness or vertigo, is very common, somewhat more so as we get older. You can induce it in yourself without any difficulty by spinning around for too long. Remember how children play "Pin the Tail on the Donkey," spinning a blindfolded playmate around and then laughing as he or she staggers toward the target. Dizziness can also come on very suddenly, with dramatic effects.

Sudden Attacks of Dizziness

A few years ago we were with a group of colleagues at a meeting in New York to evaluate some research grants. We broke for lunch and as we reassembled in the small conference room of our hotel, one of our members was missing. We waited half an hour or so and, when he still didn't appear, we called his room and got no answer. At this point we became concerned and went up and knocked on his door. A weak voice acknowledged that he was there, but that he could not get to the door to let us in. We had no idea what had happened. After being admitted with a hotel pass key, we found our colleague lying on the floor virtually unable to move. He was extraordinarily pale, extremely nauseated, and any attempt to move him, particularly to move his head, was accompanied by paroxysms of nausea and acute discomfort. He felt better with his eyes closed. When he tried to look around, his eyes made wild jerking movements. He was unable to walk because of a violent feeling that he was spinning around. In short, he felt awful and thought the end was near.

The story has a happy ending. Our colleague was having an acute disturbance of the balancing mechanisms in his inner ear. We got him to a nearby hospital, where he was given some medications to knock down his nausea and vertigo. He responded promptly to medications and he was able to fly home two days later.

The kind of disruption of the balancing mechanisms in the ears that our colleague experienced usually causes an acute attack of dizziness. The mechanisms in the two ears work together like the two engines of an airplane: if one engine suddenly loses power, then the airplane will go acutely out of balance. Dysfunction of the mechanism in one ear can occur, sometimes very suddenly, for a variety of reasons, including a possible viral infection of the inner ear or a lack of blood to the balancing mechanisms. But often the cause remains unclear.

The effect can devastate a person. As we saw with our colleague, the loss of balance, inability to move, wild jerking of the eyes (called nystagmus), nausea, and vomiting can make someone feel that he or she must be dying.

Sudden attacks of dizziness are, however, often short-lived and patients can then recover and be perfectly normal. The same remedies used for motion sickness, such as Antivert, Dramamine, or Scopolamine patches, can help these attacks of sudden dizziness. In our experience, patients with symptoms that come on very suddenly, even though they may have extreme discomfort and be extraordinarily disabled for brief periods of time, usually do not have severe long-term problems.

Repeated Attacks of Dizziness

In middle age and beyond, people can have repeated attacks of sudden dizziness that fall under an umbrella term called Meniere's Disease. These attacks begin with ringing in the ear and a decrease in hearing in that ear. After a few hours or even days, the victim will have an acute attack of dizziness. These attacks can be so severe that a person will have to lie quietly in bed until it passes. After a few hours, the dizziness subsides, but the decreased hearing and feeling of being off balance may last for days. There may be repeat attacks, with hearing getting progressively worse in the affected ear.

It is not entirely clear what produces this disease, but it appears to be related to a long-term dysfunction of the balancing mechanisms of the ear. In some patients these mechanisms accumulate too much fluid. In this case the answer is to prescribe drugs that dehydrate the body, so-called diuretics, the same kinds of drugs that often are used against high blood pressure. In severe cases, the treatment may be to slow down the balancing apparatus by partially damaging it with an antibiotic, Gentamicin. Alternatively, the nerve that brings the messages from the balancing mechanisms to the brain may be cut in a surgical procedure. After such a procedure, a person needs physical therapy to relearn how to balance properly.

Dizziness with Head Movements

For at least 10 years Anna, a charming elderly lady, experienced dizziness when she moved her head in certain ways. At night, she slept only with her right ear down. If she turned over in bed quickly, or forgot and lay down on her left side, she might have a sudden spinning sensation for two or three minutes. During the day, she could almost never look upward. Lifting her chin to look at her kitchen clock over the sink could bring on the dizziness. Sometimes the spinning was so violent that she had to grasp the sink to keep from falling.

Often older people have episodes of dizziness when they put their heads in certain positions or move their heads quickly. This problem, carrying the fancy name "benign positional vertigo," causes the most dizziness in older people.

The cause of Anna's positional vertigo is that the very small stones in her ear (the otoliths we mentioned earlier, in chapter 10) became damaged with age; some of these otoliths fell from their position and accumulated in one place when her head was in a particular position. When she turned her head, these little stones moved, and sent a false signal to her brain. Recently we tried some positional exercises to help her. She lay for a few minutes with one ear down, then a few minutes with the other down. Then we shook her head—particularly when the "bad" side was down. The idea was to shake the otoliths out of the areas where they had accumulated and back into place. You can't do these positional exercises by yourself; you need someone familiar with this form of treatment to guide you, because the exercises are not done the same way in all patients. What a doctor might do is determined, in part, by what brings on the attacks of dizziness. Properly done, treatment can be very successful. In Anna's case these maneuvers worked, and she is much more mobile than she was before—but still very cautious about looking up.

WHAT YOU CAN DO ABOUT FAINTING AND DIZZINESS: UNDERSTAND THE SIGNS

Light-headedness on standing up is a warning sign that your blood pressure may be too low and you could faint. If you notice this type of faintness repeatedly, consider having your blood pressure checked. If you are taking certain medications that can increase the likelihood of fainting, such as drugs for high blood pressure or Parkinson's disease, keep in mind that the danger time is when you stand up after lying down for a long period. Be sure to get up gradually, spending a few minutes sitting.

Dizziness that follows head movements, such as turning your head, rolling over in bed, or looking up can often be corrected with specific exercises—ask your doctor.

PART THREE

THE BRAIN AND PREVENTING AND TREATING SERIOUS PROBLEMS

CHAPTER 12

UNDERSTANDING ACUTE
MEMORY LOSS

Ron was at a Fourth of July picnic with his family. Because he was not drinking, he volunteered to go and get some more beer for the others. While driving down a country lane, he attempted to dodge a truck that was coming from the opposite direction at a high speed. His car hit a pole and he was knocked unconscious. By the time people came to his aid, he was up and walking around, but his memory was not normal. When the police arrived he was able to talk to them and give his name, but he did not know where he was or where he had been going. In the ambulance on the way to the hospital, he appeared to be alert and talked to people, but he had no memory of the picnic, or the details of the accident. Later, in the emergency room, his memory of the picnic and leaving to get the beer gradually returned. However, he had no memory of the ride to the emergency room or the discussion with doctors there. This loss of memory persisted for six or seven hours and then began to clear. To this day, however, he does not remember how he got from the site of the accident to the hospital.

A blow to the head disturbed Ron's memory. However, other things, including drugs, alcohol, and interruptions in blood supply to the brain, can also produce a sudden loss of memory. What they all have in common is that, in most instances, a person is quite normal and then something happens to the brain that disrupts the memory system in a very specific way.

HEAD INJURY AND SUDDEN LOSS OF MEMORY

Most frequently, sudden memory loss is a result of a blow to the head, as with Ron. In older people, falls and automobile accidents are the usual causes. To trigger memory loss, the blow to the head usually must be severe enough to cause at least a brief period of unconsciousness. But even people who do not get knocked out can still lose their memory of recent events, such as where they have been and what they were doing, most likely because the blow disrupts the memory-forming process before the brain has time to consolidate these events.

Of course, sudden memory loss can affect anyone, not just older individuals. It often strikes participants in contact sports, such as boxers and football players. When a football player gets knocked out on the field and a trainer runs out to tend to him, the first questions the trainer asks are, "Where are you?" "Who are you playing?" and "What's the score?" If the player answers these questions accurately, he probably is all right. Still, every so often a player can get up and walk around but be totally unable to answer these simple questions. There is no particular treatment for such loss of memory following a head injury, except to be sure that no underlying brain injury requires surgery. However, a head injury severe enough to cause a sudden loss of memory may entail subtle changes in neural function that can require weeks or months to return to normal. These may include problems with sleep and change in behavior, such as irritability or difficulty with concentration.

Repeated head injuries do not make a player more likely to be knocked out the next time, but they can lead to permanent brain damage because the brain never has time to recover completely. The great boxer Muhammad Ali exemplifies what can happen over time in extreme cases. Once as nimble with ideas and words as he was with his fists and footwork, Ali now has difficulty thinking and moving because of the many blows to the head he incurred during his boxing career.

In other instances, a single blow to the head may be severe enough to preclude full recovery. In such individuals the initial problem may be memory loss, but the long-term problems may be different. They can include difficulty concentrating, handling frustrating situations, and effectively planning one's actions.

Prevention is the most effective course of action with respect to head injury. Always wear seat belts in the car, and always wear a helmet when you are bike riding or engaging in any other sport that carries a risk of head injury.

BLOOD SUPPLY TO THE BRAIN AND SUDDEN MEMORY LOSS

Elaine was a healthy middle-aged woman, except for a history of migraine. Her headaches usually occurred two or three times a year, with a warning stage that usually consisted of flashing lights in her eyes. A severe headache would then follow, lasting for one or two days. One day, in the middle of a bridge party at her home, she realized that she didn't know where she was, whom she was with, or what was happening. At about the same time, her fellow card players began to realize that she could not keep track of the bidding. Concerned, they brought her to the hospital. Shortly after arriving, she suddenly became aware of where she was, but had no idea of how she had gotten there. The examining doctor admitted her, so that he could try to determine the cause of her problems. He decided to present her at one of the conferences held each week at the hospital to get input from other neurologists. At the conference she was her normal self—an intelligent woman with no evidence of memory problems, except that she had no recollection of the afternoon bridge party at which she had experienced a brief memory loss, a condition called a transient global amnesia. As Elaine was leaving the meeting, she was asked if she could find her way back to her room just around the corner. She replied that she would wait there, before going home, because she wanted to know what had been determined at the conference. A short while later, the physician went to her room, but she had vanished. A frantic search ensued. Eventually, the physician found Elaine in the main cafeteria having a cup of coffee. She knew who she was, but had no idea why she was in the hospital, in what room she resided, or who her physicians were. Apparently, she had had another episode of sudden memory loss. He whisked her to the electroencephalography laboratory where tests gave us insight into her particular problem. He came to the conclusion that her migraine condition was affecting the blood vessels leading to the part of the brain essential for normal memory. He treated her with a drug called Propranolol that changes the response of the blood vessels and also reduces the neurotransmitter serotonin, which appears to be involved in migraine. Elaine has had no further episodes, but she has changed one behavior: after a conference, the physicians no longer send patients to their rooms unescorted!

A temporary loss of memory can also stem from a lack of circulation of blood to the brain. This condition arises most commonly in people like Elaine who have a history of migraine headaches. Less commonly, it results from a transient ischemic attack or TIA (discussed in chapter 19, "Stroke: The Brain-Heart Connection." In both transient global amnesia and TIA, memory loss stems from a temporary decrease in blood supply to the areas of the brain responsible for taking in and retaining new information.

DRUGS AND ALCOHOL AND SUDDEN MEMORY LOSS

Excess alcohol and certain kinds of drugs also commonly cause sudden memory loss. After drinking alcohol excessively, a person's memory usually returns to normal when he or she sobers up, but gaps may remain. The individual may not remember what was said at a cocktail party or what occurred during the course of an evening, for example.

Medications can do the same thing. A popular sleeping pill, Halcion, can trigger a striking memory loss—so much so that for a period of time the British took it off the market. Many compounds used for anesthesia affect memory, as well. Just before falling asleep in the operating room, patients may carry on a conversation or babble about many things. When they awaken after surgery, they have no memory of what they said.

WHAT HAPPENS IN THE BRAIN WITH SUDDEN MEMORY LOSS

The study of sudden memory loss has produced fundamental insights into how memory mechanisms work. Initially, researchers focused their attention on people who suffered permanent brain damage that left them unable to learn new information, but still retain much of the information they had acquired previously. These studies led to the conclusion that a part of the brain called the hippocampal region is essential for learning new information. In actuality we have two hippocampal regions, one on each side of the brain. The hippocampus acts rather like a funnel—information comes into the mouth of the funnel and then has to pass through a very narrow spout (the hippocampus) in order to get to the cerebral cortex, the brain's permanent storage tank. The hippocampal region of the brain is particularly vulnerable to a temporary interruption in its blood supply. Elaine's sudden but temporary memory loss while playing bridge occurred because for a short time the blood supply was deficient to the hippocampus on both sides of her brain. Short reductions in the supply of oxygen to the brain also cause relatively brief problems with memory. For example, if a person's brain does not get enough oxygen for only a short period during a heart attack, he or she may be temporarily unable to retain new information. Infections from certain viruses also can damage the hippocampus on both sides of the brain, resulting in permanent memory difficulty. Interestingly, a sudden loss of memory does not usually occur in most people with strokes, because strokes usually involve only one side of the brain.

Individuals who experience brain damage that primarily affects the hippocampus but leaves other parts of the brain relatively unscathed can appear superficially normal, but in fact they have severe problems in learning new information. When we see such a patient in the hospital, we might introduce ourselves, discuss where they are, the day and the date, and talk about the morning news. The patient can repeat all this information to us, and so clearly understands what we are saying. However, if we leave the room and come back 15 minutes later, the patient will forget everything that we discussed. This inability to form new memories after an injury to the brain is called anterograde amnesia (after the prefix "antero" which means "forward").

Newer brain imaging techniques, particularly magnetic resonance imaging (MRI), reveal the hippocampal region with great clarity and make it possible to predict the likelihood of recovery. In a person with severe and permanent anterograde amnesia, this part of the brain will appear greatly shrunken or even absent on the MRI scan. An autopsy of such a person will show that the nerve cells in the hippocampal region on both sides of the brain have been virtually destroyed.

A sudden injury to the brain may also take away memory of events prior to the injury, as occurred with Ron. This retrograde amnesia (after the prefix "retro" which means "back") is usually short-lived, and memory of events before the injury returns over a matter of minutes or hours. Such a loss of memory is a temporary inability to recall events that were already recorded in the brain. Clearly the information is there; one just cannot bring it back.

Returning to our funnel analogy, it is as if information is kept in a temporary holding tank before passing through to the larger tank for long-term storage. This is, in fact, how the memory system of the brain works. After information is processed by the hippocampus, it goes to other parts of the brain for storage. This storage process in the brain is complex and, for a time, the new memories remain vulnerable to disruption. That is why the retrograde amnesia impairs memories of very recent events more than older ones that have been been securely stored for a long period of time.

As we discussed in chapter 1, "Maintaining Your Memory," the essential part of the memory process is the connections between nerve cells. The basic cellular unit of the brain, the nerve cell or neuron, recognizes, processes, and integrates information with hundreds of millions of other nerve cells, all working in intricately orchestrated ways. When we store memories, we change the connections between the nerve cells in the memory system. In doing so, we are probably both making new connections and strengthening existing ones. Initially the new connections are less secure, and therefore more vulnerable to disruption in the event that the brain is hurt. How these new connections are strengthened or made is a very active area of research. Once we understand how the connections between nerve cells in the memory system are strengthened, then we will know how to reinforce this process.

MEMORY LOSS RELATED TO PSYCHOLOGICAL PROBLEMS

Some people complain of memory difficulty that does not appear to be related to a true disruption of the memory system. These people appear to be in two groups, those reacting to a traumatic emotional event, and those who are faking memory problems.

In the first group, an individual having a reaction to an emotional shock, such as a woman after a rape or a soldier after a battle, might be found wandering in a confused state. Such individuals seem to lose personal knowledge about themselves, their family, their position in life, or their job. At the same time, however, they can make correct associations about events in the past that did not particularly involve them personally, such as a past presidential election. This pattern is never seen in someone who has actual brain damage to the memory system. Patients with emotional traumas as the cause of their memory difficulty can sometimes be helped by an Amytal interview. During this procedure a person is injected with a graded dose of Amytal, a short-acting drug. The physician then speaks quietly and gently with the patient to encourage recall of the emotionally traumatic events. Intact memories often return during this process. Afterward, the physician can work with the patient to help him or her adjust to the emotional problems that caused the memory loss.

The second group of individuals consists of those who are faking or malingering. Such individuals may show up in a distant location claiming to not know who they are and being unable to remember their family or background. They do, however, have accurate knowledge of what is going on around them and are able to pick up and learn new information in a manner that is quite normal. This pattern of defect in memory is virtually never seen in people who have memory loss due to brain damage. Almost always a hidden precipitating event, such as embezzlement from a bank or desertion from the military, eventually comes to light. Malingerers may be very hard to detect. Recently, specific memory tests have been developed to differentiate true memory loss from this artificial problem with memory.

RESEARCH IN SUDDEN PROBLEMS WITH MEMORY

Sudden loss of memory results from a variety of injuries to the brain. Even though the causes may vary, it is possible that the treatment designed for one condition may apply to others, including sudden memory loss. Many pharmaceutical companies are competing to develop drugs that will alter how the brain responds to an injury, including head injury, stroke, and lack of oxygen to the brain. Several drugs have been developed that are quite effective in experimental animals and are now being tried in people.

WHAT YOU CAN DO ABOUT SUDDEN CHANGES IN MEMORY: PREVENTION IS THE KEY

The best way to prevent sudden changes in memory is to avoid, if possible, the situations that lead to them. Protect yourself against head injury by buckling your seat belt in the car and wear a helmet for bicycling and other sports where head injury is a possibility; avoid excessive amounts of alcohol. Check the advice for improving balance and coordination in chapter 10, "How to Keep Your Balance—Literally."

If you do experience an unexpected, unexplained loss of memory, call your doctor. Early recognition and treatment can shorten the duration of symptoms and help them to be less severe.

CHAPTER 13

ACUTE CONFUSION AND HOW TO PREVENT IT

Recently, Marilyn went to visit an older man, Charles, a lifelong friend who had undergone surgery the previous day. Marilyn found Charles sitting up in bed, very alert, talking away at a great rate. "What a remarkable recovery for a person in his eighties," Marilyn thought. It soon became apparent, however, that Charles was making very little sense. He was talking to his wife, who had been dead for several years. Then he described an episode that had happened to one of his children many years before, as if it had happened just that day. He seemed quite uncertain about who Marilyn was, remembering her as a child, even though she had seen him the night before his surgery. Marilyn was so upset about this behavior that she called Charles' son, a surgeon at another hospital, to report what she was observing. To her surprise, the son said, "Don't worry about it, we see this kind of confusion lots of the time, especially in older people after surgery!"

Marilyn decided to follow her older friend's progress, and she went back every few hours over the next few days to see how he was doing. Charles quickly recovered physically, but his confusion went on day and night. His sleeping pattern was markedly altered: He stayed awake talking much of the night, sometimes quite agitatedly, then dozed during the day. At times the slightest stimulus, such as the lights being turned on in the room, caused him to sit bolt upright in bed. He accused nurses of all kinds of things they had not done. At times he got very angry, and at other times, such as when he talked about his deceased wife, he became upset and very sad. After three or four days, his confusion slowly cleared, although it gradually worsened again toward the evening hours each day. By the end of the week, except for a few episodes early in the evening, he was back to his normal self, but with very little memory of his recent cognitive problems.

Charles had many of the symptoms typical of a common problem called acute confusion. Acute confusion is extremely common among older persons, particularly those in hospitals and nursing homes. We are often asked to evaluate such patients because the symptoms of acute confusion not only interfere with the treatment of other diseases that the patient may have, but also lead to longer hospital stays. Fortunately, acute confusion can be prevented and treated.

What Causes Acute Confusion?

Confusion occurs mainly in three situations. In the first, a person has normal mental function but becomes confused because of some external factor, such as medication or surgery. For such people, confusion is a temporary condition. In the second situation, confusion can accompany a sudden brain injury from a stroke, the side effects of a heart attack, or a head injury. Recovery depends on the extent of the injury to the brain. The third situation, the most common one, occurs when someone has an abnormality in brain function and an additional problem causes them to get worse suddenly. Such individuals may have had a previous injury to the brain, such as a stroke, or a progressive disease of the brain, such as Alzheimer's disease. Many things can tip these people over into confusion—a general infection such as a urinary tract infection or pneumonia, dehydration on a hot day, or even a change in environment. Often several apply to the same person.

Confusion and Medications

Almost any medication can cause confusion in an older person. Unfortunately, in our society, patients often have several physicians, each of whom might prescribe medications for the particular problem with which he or she is dealing. The heart doctor, the bladder doctor, and the brain doctor each gives his or her own medication. Thus a patient may enter the hospital taking six or seven different medications, several of which can cause confusion. Sleeping medications, heart medicine, and medicines for high blood pressure are particularly likely to cause confusion. A commonly overlooked cause of confusion is dehydration. Diuretics (medications that are designed to promote the loss of water from the body, often given to reduce the strain on an overworked heart) can make dehydration even worse.

Confusion during Hospitalization

Besides issues of medication and dehydration, other factors can place an older person at increased risk for acute confusion during a hospital stay. These include visual or hearing impairment, sleep deprivation, and immobility.

Confusion following Surgery and Anesthesia

As many as 30 percent of older patients will have the type of post-surgical symptoms that Charles experienced. Symptoms of confusion make these patients' care very difficult. They may try to pull out the IV lines that have been inserted in their arm, try to get out of bed unassisted, or refuse to take medications. Thus confusion after surgery generally results in increased complications, longer stays in intensive care units, and increased hospital costs. It is not entirely clear what causes this condition, but most physicians feel that the culprit is general anesthesia. Anesthetics appear to affect the brains of older people differently from those of younger people, for reasons that we will discuss below.

Confusion Accompanying a Sudden Brain Injury

Confusion often accompanies a fall or other blow to the head. But confusion can also occur after a stroke or a heart attack, which may have deprived the brain of sufficient blood for a brief period of time. In these situations, the duration of the confusion and the ultimate outcome depend on the severity of the injury to the brain.

Confusion in Someone with a Previous Brain Injury or Disease

Individuals who have had a previous stroke, or who are in the later stages of Parkinson's disease or any stage of Alzheimer's disease, are highly susceptible to confusion. When a person in one of these groups suddenly becomes confused, it is a tip-off that something else is going on. In some instances, the same factors that produce confusion in a normal person—medications or a fall—also do so in someone with a previous brain disorder. But, in addition, conditions that would not produce confusion in someone who was previously normal—pneumonia, a urinary tract infection, dehydration—may produce confusion in someone with a previous brain disorder.

Confusion Related to Environmental Change

Medical factors aren't the only source of acute confusion. Individuals with or without a previous brain disorder often find changes disorienting, especially when the structure of everyday life seem to crumble. Someone who leaves home, whether for a short stay in the hospital or a more permanent move to a retirement community or nursing home, may feel lost in an empty and alien world. Familiar objects are no longer there. Daily routines change and meals happen at different times. Familiar people are no longer around as much, and unfamiliar people take their place. This is particularly true when an older person enters a hospital. This is an extreme form of a phenomenon we all experience, when we wake up in a strange place and for a few moments are not entirely sure where we are. The problem becomes worse when someone suffers a degree of sensory deprivation because of decreased hearing, vision, or both. A change in environment, such as a move to a nursing home, may trigger this sort of confusion every day or every time a person awakens from a nap.

WHAT HAPPENS TO THE BRAIN DURING CONFUSION?

Confusion occurs when the different parts of the brain do not function together well, and thus do not process information correctly. Charles, for example, had problems keeping things organized in time. He thought Marilyn was still a child, even though seeing her should have been sufficient to dispel that idea. When Charles thought of his wife, he remembered her as still being alive, even though she had been dead for several years. At times, he was too alert and any sound would arouse him even more. His brain apparently couldn't quiet down or modulate the incoming stimuli in a normal way. In instances of acute confusion, no specific part of the brain has been irreversibly injured; instead, different parts of the brain interact in abnormal ways. Medicines such as Risperdal or Haldol can can calm down people with acute confusion and prevent them from harming themselves or others. Once the precipitating factors are removed, mental abilities gradually return to normal.

How to Keep Confusion at Bay on the Medical Side

The best way to handle confusion is to prevent it from happening. Patients and family members should keep abreast of any medications being taken. Almost any medication, but particularly combinations of medication, can produce confusion. Older people process chemical agents differently from younger people, and there can be considerable individual variation in how they handle medications. If possible, people should start a new medication at a low dose and then gradually increase the amount. By the same token, people should try to avoid starting two medications at the same time. Otherwise, if a person becomes confused, it will take extra time to figure out whether one of the two medications or the combination of both is causing the problem. Sleep aids, such as Dalmane, Seconal, Halcion, or Ambien, lead the list of medications that can produce confusion.

To prevent dehydration, it is important to encourage older people to drink enough fluids, particularly those who take diuretics for their heart. When they can't drink enough, intravenous fluids should be considered, even if an individual is living at home.

Because general anesthesia has such unpredictable effects on older people, surgeons use it less frequently than they used to. Instead, common surgeries, such as those for prostate cancer or hip and knee replacements, are now largely done with local injections of anesthetic agents that merely block pain at a particular location. This results in much less postoperative confusion, fewer complications, and shorter stays in the hospital.

Steps that Family and Friends Can Take

Individuals helping to care for older people can do a great deal to prevent acute confusion from developing by being aware of its causes and watching for any sign of them. Moreover, the steps necessary to minimize confusion are simple things that take only a few minutes several times a day. These include such things as keeping people aware of their surroundings, helping them to be as physically active as possible, and being sure they drink enough water and get as much sleep as they can. Many simple measures can minimize unnecessary additional illness and hospitalization. (See "What You Can Do about Acute Confusion," page 162).

How to Treat Confusion Once It Occurs

Preventing confusion is vital because the ability to treat it is limited. The first step is to try and remove the cause of the problem, which often must be done by trial and error. If this doesn't work, it is often necessary to use medication to keep the confused patient, and those nearby, safe.

Reducing Medications

If a patient is confused, all medicines should be suspect. But medicines that have been added recently or for which the dosage has been changed are the likeliest culprits. Sometimes, however, a medication a patient has been taking for a long time causes difficulties. Switching between name brand and generic versions of a medication may also be a problem because of subtle differences between the two. A patient's physician may have to go back to square one, removing as many medications as possible, and starting all over again, adding one at a time.

Adding Medications

Paradoxically, when agitated behavior threatens to harm the patient or others, it may be necessary to add further medications. Drugs such as Haldol, Risperdal, Clozapine, or Olanzepine can sometimes help calm the patient. But these medications should be used in very low doses and for as short a time as possible.

Responding to the Patient with Confusion

In the long term, altering the way one interacts with the patient or making changes in the environment work better than relying on medications. The first and most important thing is to ensure that the patient receives medical care as quickly as possible. In addition, sudden confusion can be extremely frightening to the patient as well as to relatives and friends. But if properly treated, confused individuals are likely to return to their previous level of mental ability. It is also important to recognize that the patient cannot control the confused behavior; friends and family shouldn't take what they say or do personally. Lastly, a person who has had one episode of sudden confusion is likely to have another, particularly if medicines are responsible. In these days of managed health care, when continuity of care is in peril, it is unfortunately up to the patient (or to a vigilant family member) to inform the appropriate physicians about past episodes of confusion and the need be particularly careful when introducing new medications.

RESEARCH IN ACUTE CONFUSION

How well someone does after an episode of acute confusion depends on how the brain functioned beforehand, what caused the confusion, and how it is treated. More progress has been made in preventing acute confusion than in reversing it. This is, in part, because acute confusion usually has more than one cause and it can take a great deal of trial and error to determine the correct therapy. The problem that is most easily reversible, but the hardest to detect by observation, is dehydration. At present, physicians identify dehydration by detecting increased concentrations of chemicals in the blood. It ought to be possible to do this with a simpler test that can be used at home. In addition, researchers need to develop drugs that will shorten the duration and lessen the severity of confusion once it occurs.

WHAT YOU CAN DO ABOUT ACUTE CONFUSION: CONSISTENCY IS KEY

Family and friends are one of the first lines of defense in preventing confusion. Since confusion is so often a reaction to change, a little advance planning can help keep things consistent. For a temporary hospitalization, for example, check to make sure the room will be well lighted. Try to make the environment familiar, bringing to the hospital a few items from home; if the move is permanent, try furnishing the new apartment with treasured pieces. A large calendar and a clearly visible clock can help keep an individual grounded in the correct the date and time. An optimal sound level is also important; a room that is too noisy can be distracting, while too much quiet may cross the border into sensory deprivation. Turning on a television or radio from time to time can provide some stimulation. It is also important to be aware of any difficulties with hearing or vision, and to be sure that the usual hearing and visual aids are available.

Whether in the hospital or at an old home or new one, if at all possible try to preserve daily rituals such as taking walks, playing cards, or watching favorite television shows together. Maybe even start a few new rituals as well. A daily walk can do wonders; if patients cannot get out of bed, then simple exercises to get their arms and legs moving are helpful. Physical activity in itself may help sharpen the brain; it also provides a way to interact with others and to stay aware of the details in the environment. Regular mental stimulation, such as a discussion of past or current events, can also keep a person properly oriented.

Whatever the living situation, improving sleep will reduce the likelihood that confusion will occur. Simple things such as a warm drink at night (milk or herbal tea), relaxation tapes, or music can go a long way to improving sleep.

In the hospital, reducing emotional stress as much as possible will also help prevent confusion. When in a hospital, people like and need to be informed about what is happening. They need to know when they are going to have procedures done or if another doctor is going to see them, and why. These explanations can go a long way to lessen the anxieties that inevitably accompany a hospital stay. Even in the best hospitals, schedules go awry and things don't always happen as expected. If possible, a friend or family member should act as a patient advocate for an older person, making sure that he or she knows what is supposed to happen when, and acting as unofficial liaison between the patient and the medical staff to ensure that surprises are kept to a minimum.

Older people who are experiencing a change in living situation, such as moving to a retirement community or going into a nursing home, also need considerable reassurance.

They have a genuine feeling of loss—after all, they have lost their homes and, in a sense, their past, since memories are so often evoked by association. They need to be reassured that their financial affairs are being properly handled, that their family and children have not abandoned them, and that people will care about them and for them.

CHAPTER 14

DEALING WITH ALZHEIMER'S DISEASE AND OTHER DEMENTIAS

A friend of ours recently began to tell us about her mother, Sarah. "Her memory is really terrible now," she said. Sarah was widowed in her early 70s but remained very independent and active and traveled widely. She took responsibility for all aspects of her daily life, including handling her taxes, and making all the plans for her many trips. One day, our friend found Sarah, then 82, looking over the income tax forms in tears. "I just can't do this anymore," she said. Our friend thought nothing of it at the time, and arranged for someone to help her mother with her taxes. But Sarah continued to pay her own bills and handle her daily activities with little problem.

Over time, however, her memory began to get worse and worse. She started to forget stories she'd been told, and she began repeating herself, apparently having forgotten that she had said the same thing earlier. This happened so gradually that our friend did not notice how much difficulty her mother was having with memory. It was only when her mother got lost on a trip that she realized how serious the situation had become. Sarah had to fly to Miami to join a cruise. She arrived in the Miami airport and realized that she did not remember the name of the cruise line and had forgotten the documents that would have provided the information. Our friend received a frightened phone call from her mother and fortunately had the itinerary with the necessary information. But she realized that something was seriously wrong and sought a medical evaluation for her mother. The results indicated that Sarah had Alzheimer's disease (AD).

Marilyn sees people like Sarah in her clinic all the time. She is often involved in giving families a diagnosis and providing guidance about treatment throughout the illness. Because Alzheimer's disease, a form of dementia, is such a common disorder, she is also frequently asked for advice by friends and colleagues seeking help with family members.

Ten years ago we could make the diagnosis and do little else. Now there are some treatments we can offer, and we are increasingly optimistic about the possibilities of early diagnosis and newer approaches to treatment.

The word "dementia" describes a condition in which a person has lost so much mental ability that he or she can no longer function normally. Many things can cause dementia, but the most common is Alzheimer's disease. It produces dementia because it attacks the parts of the brain responsible for mental abilities such as memory, language, and spatial skill. Alzheimer's disease is named for a German physician, Alois Alzheimer, who saw a middle-aged woman having increasing difficulty with her memory. Over time she began to have trouble expressing herself and understanding others, and gradually all of her mental faculties became impaired. Ultimately, she was unable to care for herself at all. She developed pneumonia and died at the age of 51.

A close colleague of Alzheimer's, a physician named Nissl, had just developed a new way of examining brain tissue with a stain that contained silver. Different stains bring out different aspects of a tissue's structure, and when Alzheimer examined the brain tissue of his patient at autopsy with Nissl's new stain, the silver revealed two abnormalities that had never been described before. Alzheimer called them plaques and tangles, and scientists still use those terms today. In 1907, Alzheimer published an article describing his patient and the changes that he saw in her brain tissue after she died. Shortly afterward, people began using the name Alzheimer's disease to refer to patients whose mental impairment followed a similar course and who had similar plaques and tangles in their brains.

Because Alzheimer's patient was relatively young (only 51), people thought that Alzheimer's disease only affected people under the age of 65. Not until the mid-1970s did scientists realize that many elderly people who had progressive and irreversible difficulty with memory and other mental abilities showed the same pattern of plaques and tangles in their brains. Prior to that, the belief was that most of these individuals became demented because the blood supply to their brain was restricted by hardening of the arteries. Others referred to these individuals as being senile, which is just another way of saying that someone is elderly and has dementia.

It soon became clear that most elderly people with dementia had Alzheimer's disease and that the total number of such individuals over the age of 65 was very large. About 1 in every 10 people in their 70s has the disease. And the numbers go up dramatically as people get older—at least 1 in every 4 individuals over 85 has Alzheimer's disease. As of 2001, some 3 million people in the United States had the disease. If nothing changes, due to the aging of the population that number could be as high as 4 million by 2025.

HOW DOES ALZHEIMER'S DISEASE BEGIN?

Progressive problems with memory are usually the first sign of Alzheimer's disease. Since the disease comes on in such a slow and subtle manner, the initial symptoms look just like the normal difficulties we all have from time to time—misplacing our keys, forgetting a message someone gave us, having trouble remembering where we parked the car. The difference is that for the person with Alzheimer's disease these problems get worse and worse over time. Problems that only happened once every few months begin happening every week or every day. In addition, the person in the early phase of Alzheimer's disease often has difficulty recalling a logical sequence of events. When a brain-healthy person loses her keys, she can usually reconstruct what happened and say, "Aha, now I remember what I did." For the person in the early phase of Alzheimer's disease, the absence of that "Aha!" moment is often the first sign that something is really wrong.

By the time someone with Alzheimer's disease is having this much memory difficulty, he or she is also usually having trouble with planning and organizing. For example, a person who was always conscientious about her checkbook may no longer be able to keep a balance. A person who regularly planned family trips or kept the accounts may begin having trouble with these familiar tasks. An accomplished cook may become confused while putting together a complicated meal, forget favorite recipes or ingredients, or overcook or burn food.

Regardless of whether the difficulties are in the areas of memory, planning and organization, or the like, in Alzheimer's disease they come on gradually. If someone develops problems in these areas overnight, the likely cause is a stroke rather than Alzheimer's disease. In fact, the problems in Alzheimer patients come on so gradually that only in retrospect can one guess when they began. In the case of Sarah, Alzheimer's disease was certainly well under way by the time she felt overwhelmed by the prospect of doing her taxes. Deciding when Alzheimer's has begun depends on recognizing subtle changes in the experience and behavior of the individual in question.

A very small number of individuals do not have significant memory difficulty during the earliest phase of Alzheimer's disease.

Their symptoms begin instead with either spatial or language difficulty. Spatial difficulty usually shows up as a loss of coordination that hinders them in leisure sports activities, such as golf or bowling. People who experience these symptoms often feel as if their vision is deteriorating; they go to the eye doctor over and over trying to find a prescription for glasses that will help. But the deterioration is in the way their brains handle information about objects in space, not in their eyes. Eventually these people develop substantial problems with memory, planning, and language, like other patients with Alzheimer's disease.

The people who begin with language difficulty act differently in the early phase of disease than those with spatial or memory difficulty. The former generally begin by having trouble finding the words to express what they want to say. Soon other aspects of language become affected, and individuals start to struggle with writing and reading and with understanding what other people are saying.

Just as the individual who begins with spatial difficulty sooner or later develops other Alzheimer's symptoms, the person with a "language presentation" of Alzheimer's disease eventually loses ground with memory, planning, and other cognitive skills.

Regardless of the nature of the earliest symptoms, the course of disease varies widely among individuals. Some people can become completely dependent on others for the basic activities of daily living, such as eating and dressing, within five years; others may take 15 years to reach the same degree of dependency. The reasons for this variability remain a mystery.

How Is Alzheimer's Disease Diagnosed?

There is no specific test for Alzheimer's disease, and therefore diagnosis takes several steps. The first step is to determine if a person really does have a significant, progressive memory problem by talking with a family member or close friend about the changes that have occurred and the time course of the changes. The physician needs to get a clear idea of what the person was like many years ago, in order to assess what changes have developed over time.

Neuropsychological tests are then carried out to compare a person's performance with those of a similar age and educational background. The earliest abnormalities found on these cognitive tests usually involve memory, particularly the ability to learn and recall new information, and in an area called "executive function"—the ability to plan and execute complex acts. The pattern of change on cognitive testing can help distinguish Alzheimer's disease from other causes of dementia.

The third step is to look for diseases other than Alzheimer's, particularly ones that can be treated, that might progressively erode cognitive function. Ruling out other diseases requires a physical or neurological examination, as well as standard laboratory tests. For example, people with evidence of a gradually progressive decline in memory are given tests to rule out a vitamin deficiency, such as vitamin B12 deficiency. They also undergo an array of standard laboratory tests to check for problems with the thyroid, liver, and the like, which also can cause problems with mental ability. Finally, an imaging study of the brain, either a CT or MRI, can demonstrate the presence of two treatable conditions: normal pressure hydrocephalus or subdural hematoma (see chapter 16, "Treatable Dementias").

What Goes Wrong in Alzheimer's Disease?

Alzheimer's disease is an example of what happens when a brain system degenerates; its progress reflects the complexity of brain structures and mental abilities. The first part of the brain that is affected in most people is the hippocampus and surrounding regions, which are essential for normal memory. Plaques and tangles, just like the ones that Alois Alzheimer saw under his microscope, slowly form in the hippocampus and surrounding structures, causing the nerve cells to die. Over time, the plaques and tangles spread to other brain regions, and nerve cells start to die there as well. What is remarkable is that the affected brain regions involve complex mental abilities—memory, planning, language, and spatial skill. Brain regions that process more basic functions, such as touch, hearing, and breathing, remain unaffected.

The Underlying Mechanism

Our ideas about the mechanism and possible approach to treatment relate to the plaques and tangles. The plaques that Alois Alzheimer first saw in the brains of people with Alzheimer's disease contain a specific protein, known as amyloid. The brain constantly makes and breaks down amyloid, as it does many other substances. In Alzheimer's disease, something has gone awry with both the production and breakdown of amyloid. Small, abnormal pieces of amyloid accumulate and form the plaques. These abnormal pieces are thought to be toxic to nerve cells.

The discovery of three genes that cause Alzheimer's disease in people under the age of 60 helped to clarify this picture. Each of these genes makes the brain produce an increased amount of abnormal amyloid, which damages nerve cells and evokes an inflammatory response. Using genetic engineering techniques, scientists are now able to track this process in the brains of mice. In these experiments, mice receive one of the three culprit genes. Afterwards they develop excess amounts of exactly the same form of amyloid that accumulates in the human brain in Alzheimer's disease. More important, these mice experience memory difficulties: their ability to navigate a standard maze test begins to fail. Thus, "Alzheimer mice" are invaluable for testing approaches to treatment. Further animal experiments can point the way to new treatments by providing a better understanding of how both normal and abnormal amyloid act in the brain.

The tangles also contain a specific protein, tau. It is not clear what role this protein plays in the basic mechanism of Alzheimer's disease.

Genetics and Alzheimer's Disease

Every relative of a person with Alzheimer's disease has to wonder what role genetics plays in it. "Since my mother has Alzheimer's, will I or my children get it?" The answer depends primarily on the age at which a person developed Alzheimer's disease. If Alzheimer's developed before the age of 60, then some of the family members likely carry one of the abnormal genes that, when present, always causes the disease. Fortunately, this early onset occurs in only about 2 percent of the people with Alzheimer's disease. In these cases, families should seek genetic counseling to decide if they wish to see if they carry one of the three abnormal genes.

For most people, however, the answer is more complicated. At least one gene has been identified as increasing the risk of developing Alzheimer's disease, but not invariably causing it. Carrying a particular form of this gene known as APOE-4 increases the risk of Alzheimer's disease about fourfold. However, another form of this gene, APOE-2 actually decreases one's risk. This suggests that most people have sets of genes, some of which increase the risk and some of which decrease the risk of Alzheimer's disease.

Except for the rare families who develop Alzheimer's at a younger age, no genetic test for the disease exists. For all other families the question is one of increased risk. Scientists studying people with memory loss are performing tests to try to identify these possible "risk genes." We do not think this research will or should lead to a routine test of the risk of the disease. It is not useful for a person to know that he or she is at increased risk for a disease with no satisfactory treatment. Our advice will change, however, when better treatments become available, particularly those that either prevent or slow the progress of Alzheimer's disease. When this happens, patients who know they are at risk will be able to take appropriate measures, just as people who have an increased risk for a heart attack stop smoking and work hard to keep their cholesterol levels low.

Treatment of Alzheimer's Disease

The major drugs developed over the last 15 years for treatment of Alzheimer's disease evolved from findings obtained from autopsies of Alzheimer's patients. Autopsy studies revealed that the neurotransmitter acetylcholine, a chemical prevalent in parts of the brain involved in memory function, was greatly reduced in the brains of those with AD. This finding inspired the hope that increasing this chemical could stem or reverse the effects of AD. The first acetylcholine booster to be evaluated was physostigmine. This drug slows cognitive decline a little, but it has significant side effects, particularly gastrointestinal symptoms such as diarrhea, nausea, and vomiting. The modest success of physostigmine sparked a search for other, less toxic compounds. The FDA has approved four drugs for the treatment of Alzheimer's disease in the United States: Cognex, Aricept, Exelon, and Reminyl. All of them elevate acetylcholine. Cognex was the first of these drugs to win approval. However, it must be taken four times a day and, more importantly, it produces significant side effects, such as stomach upset and abnormalities of liver function, that require weekly blood tests for the first four months of treatment. Cognex now has largely been replaced by the other three, particularly Aricept. Aricept can be taken once per day and has fewer side effects than Cognex; because Exelon and Reminyl are newer, less is known about how well they work.

These medications all raise levels of acetylcholine in the brain. Although they treat the symptoms of Alzheimer's disease, they do not alter the disease's mechanism or its progression. Still, they can lead to temporary improvement. They may prove to be more useful in those in the later stages, modifying abnormal behaviors such as agitation and aggression.

We recommend Aricept for our patients, starting with a low dose and then increasing it if we can. The limiting factor is usually the gastrointestinal symptoms (nausea, vomiting, and diarrhea). Aricept seems to work for about a year and then may wear off. At that time we try either Exelon or Reminyl.

Studies suggest that a more readily available substance, vitamin E, slows the progression of Alzheimer's disease, presumably by slowing the destruction of nerve cells. A two-year study of vitamin E in a group of people with moderately severe Alzheimer's disease used high doses of vitamin E, 2,000 IU a day, which is more than 60 times the recommended daily allowance of 30 IU a day. Vitamin E improved, by about 25 percent, these people's ability to bathe, dress, handle money, and do other routine chores. Lower doses of vitamin E have not yet been studied, but the high doses produced few side effects. We generally recommend a dose of 1,000 IU of vitamin E per day to our patients.

There is also some evidence that nonsteroidal anti-inflammatory drugs (NSAIDs) may be beneficial for Alzheimer's patients. NSAIDs include ibuprofen (Motrin, Advil, or Nuprin) and naproxen (Aleve). Interest in these drugs was sparked by a study of Alzheimer's disease patients which showed that patients taking NSAIDs experienced a later onset of symptoms, less severe symptoms, and a slower progression of memory loss. NSAIDs seem to dampen the inflammation triggered by the abnormal amyloid accumulations in the brains of Alzheimer's patients.

As discussed in chapter 2, "Nutrition for the Brain: Food, Fuel, and Protection," some people have claimed that the herbal preparation ginkgo biloba helps fight Alzheimer's disease. Like Cognex, Aricept, and Exelon, ginkgo may improve cognition in those with mild or moderate Alzheimer's disease. Its major advantage may be its lack of side effects; there is no evidence that it prevents or cures Alzheimer's disease.

WHEN TO TREAT EARLY ALZHEIMER'S DISEASE

Even though the current measures are not very effective, it is important to start treatment for Alzheimer's disease as early as possible in its course. That is because when nerve cells die there is as yet no way to make them regrow. That's why we recommend that our Alzheimer's patients take at least Aricept or Exelon and vitamin E.

Sarah, our friend's mother, was treated with Aricept and vitamin E for three months. Her memory and other mental abilities were evaluated before she was treated and then again three months later. Her daughter was very pleased to see that she seemed to be more "with it." She seemed to be repeating herself less often and was more alert. The change wasn't dramatic, but it gave everyone hope that the medications were doing something, so they were continued for a year. Her test scores declined a little bit over that time, but clearly she had not declined as fast as she had been before taking the medications.

PREVENTION OF ALZHEIMER'S DISEASE

The common hormone estrogen has become an intriguing candidate for the prevention and treatment of Alzheimer's disease. Some evidence indicates that women taking estrogen develop Alzheimer's disease at a lower rate than those who do not, suggesting that estrogen may also help protect the brain and thus reduce the risk of Alzheimer's disease. When women ask whether they should take estrogen to prevent Alzheimer's disease, we suggest that they do, unless they have a strong family history of breast cancer (high estrogen levels also being linked to breast cancer). However, at the present time no definitive evidence shows that estrogen alters the course of Alzheimer's disease, once it starts.

Recently, researchers have shown that people taking a class of drugs called statins, which lower the levels of cholesterol in the blood, were less likely to have Alzheimer's disease. These studies were done by comparing large numbers of people, some taking statins and some not. The next step will be to treat people ahead of time and see if statins make any difference. Such studies are in the planning phase. We do not know enough yet to recommend statins to people with normal cholesterol levels.

BEHAVIORAL PROBLEMS IN ALZHEIMER'S DISEASE

Even though people with Alzheimer's disease are getting slowly worse over time, external events such as stress, fatigue, and a superimposed illness, like the flu, can all make symptoms temporarily much worse.

Depression

It is common for people in the early phase of Alzheimer's disease to seem less interested in things than they used to be. For example, they may withdraw from a conversation among several people or show less interest in what other family members or friends are doing. Sometimes this apathy is mistaken for depression. Depression can also occur in the early phase of Alzheimer's disease. Differentiating between depression and the apathy of Alzheimer's disease often requires careful questioning. A person who is depressed has a constellation of symptoms, including a sad mood for a significant period of time, a change in sleep pattern (either increased or decreased sleep), a change in eating pattern (either increased or decreased appetite), trouble concentrating, and feelings of hopelessness.

Depression in Alzheimer's patients should be treated, because a person who is demented will have much more trouble thinking clearly if he or she is also depressed. Because multiple medications can easily interact in problematic ways, the physician who treats the depression should preferably have experience with Alzheimer's disease. Years ago, the only medicines for the treatment of depression were likely to cause increased confusion in Alzheimer's patients because they reduced acetylcholine, one of the chemicals important for normal memory function, which is already low in people with Alzheimer's. Fortunately, some newer antidepressants do not have this side effect and have fewer side effects overall. Most fall into the class of drugs called SSRI's (selective serotonin reuptake inhibitors). We prefer SSRI's that are eliminated from the body in a day or so, such as Paxil. That period is long enough that problems will not arise if the person misses a dose, but it is short enough so that the drug will not linger in the body if troubling side effects do occur. None of these medications is without side effects, but sometimes the side effects can be used to advantage. For example, some antidepressants may cause sleepiness, which may be helpful for a depressed patient who has trouble sleeping.

Some people with Alzheimer's disease become paranoid or unusually suspicious of others. Most commonly, they believe that people are stealing from them. This may be because they are very forgetful and misplace things on an almost daily basis. If this suspiciousness interferes substantially with their daily activities, it can be treated. But it is important not to make these individuals even more suspicious by asking them to take a pill that they do not know anything about. In order to be honest with patients and, at the same time, not cause additional problems, we usually say that the medicine will help them feel more relaxed or help them sleep at night, both of which are true. Of course, we tell relatives exactly what we are doing.

The Family's Role

Because Alzheimer's disease affects a person's ability to think, it has implications for the whole family. A family member usually becomes the primary caregiver and must pay careful attention to the adjustment of roles. For example, if the patient cannot balance his checkbook, or remember where he put the Social Security check that came in the mail, or handle complicated financial planning, his spouse or a child has to take over this role. Patients sometimes make serious financial mistakes that cost them and their entire family dearly. Likewise, a person who cannot remember to take medication on a regular basis needs supervision. If someone is becoming forgetful while cooking, he or she may leave pots unattended on the stove and cause a fire or become ill from not eating properly.

Driving is the most sensitive and complicated issue of them all. We always ask caregivers if they have ridden in a car with the patient recently and if they feel the patient is driving safely. Often we are told that the person with AD has begun to limit driving to the immediate area around home and times of low traffic, and that on those occasions, they are driving safely. However, sometimes other family members have decided not to drive with the patient because they feel unsafe. This may be because no one wants to ask the patient to stop driving, and they want us to speak for them. When we do this, we always do it with the family and patient together. Because people with Alzheimer's disease are forgetful, it may be necessary to write a prescription, saying, "Do not drive."

Alzheimer's disease also takes a heavy emotional toll on the patient's family. Support groups can help families cope. Other people who have lived through the same situation can often suggest ways to handle a particular problem. They have likely experienced the same emotions and thus can be more supportive than anyone else. The national Alzheimer Association can provide information about how to contact the support group in your area.

THE PROGRESSION OF ALZHEIMER'S DISEASE

As the symptoms of Alzheimer's disease progress, they slowly get worse. In addition, new problems develop. Memory for recent events deteriorates to the point where it is almost nonexistent. Families of Alzheimer's sufferers often say that first their relative could not remember from week to week, then from day to day, and then from minute to minute. Likewise, planning and organization become very impaired, so that tasks need to be broken down into individual steps. For example, asking an Alzheimer's patient to prepare potatoes to be boiled may be overwhelming. One has to break the task down into single steps, such as peeling the potatoes, then putting the potatoes in a pot, and then putting water in the pot. A problem that first manifested itself as getting lost in unfamiliar areas while driving now means getting lost on a walk around the block.

Patients also begin to have substantial problems with language. At this point it's best to speak to them in short, simple sentences. They also have increasing trouble expressing themselves and spend a considerable amount of time trying to find the right words. This slowness can frustrate the listener, who may become impatient and have a tendency to interrupt.

Behavioral problems don't develop in all individuals, but when they do, they can create havoc. Patients may wander around their homes, particularly at night, or want to walk outside, where they may get lost. Often a neighbor will spot the wanderer and bring him or her back home. Some individuals begin pacing and can't be persuaded to sit down until they have walked around enough to be tired. Others see things that aren't there or think people are doing things that they aren't doing. Usually these hallucinations and delusions have some basis in reality, such as shadows across a room that the person misinterprets. These problems are particularly likely to occur at night. There may be a reversal of the normal sleep patterns, with patients up most of the night. Most of the time these behavioral problems can be reduced by changes in the way one interacts with the individuals, or by changing the person's schedule of activities. Otherwise, Aricept or Exelon may help alleviate these problems.

Marilyn first evaluated Peter, a former salesman, when he was mildly impaired. As his disease progressed, she began to worry about his wife, because she had so little help caring for him at home. Marilyn suggested that she reduce this burden by having him go to a day care program a few days a week. However, Peter was resistant. At her suggestion, his wife told him that the day care program needed help and would hire him to work several days a week. He agreed to go but insisted on seeing his weekly check. The day care program designed a check that had his name on it but could not be cashed. Peter then went happily to "work" three times a week. After "working" for several months, Peter decided that he needed a raise.

So, of course, the day care program increased the amount of money on the "check" and Peter continues to go happily.

NURSING HOME CARE

In the late phase of the disease, patients are totally dependent on others for their care, including eating and hygiene. People caring for them need to use very simple words and sentences, and need to be very observant of the patients' responses in order to figure out what they want and how they feel.

At some point, family members must decide whether the person with Alzheimer's disease can be taken care of properly at home. In some situations this is possible, but requires obtaining reliable outside help. The alternative is nursing home placement. In our experience, family members often resist this, because they feel the patient will be unhappy and poorly cared for. In fact, if a nursing home is a good one (and there are many) the patient will receive good care and may benefit greatly from the company of others and daily programs that are geared to his or her level of ability. In addition, the family member is freed to spend quality time with the patient, rather than getting exhausted by the quantity of time required for hour-to-hour care.

Nursing home care is expensive, however, costing as much as $50,000 per year. Sometimes careful financial planning can help a family tackle this problem. For example, many people have long-term health care insurance to meet this contingency. Alternatively, families can shift resources so that a person will be eligible for Medicaid. If nursing home care is simply not an option (and for many it is not), other types of care are often available. (See "What You Can Do about Alzheimer's Disease and Other Dementias: Resources and Options for Caregivers," page 185.)

RESEARCH AND FUTURE TREATMENTS FOR ALZHEIMER'S DISEASE

It is imperative that ways to prevent and treat this disease be found. If prevention efforts could delay the average onset of the disease by only five years, it would have enormous impact. If the sharp increase in numbers of cases could be delayed until people reached age 90, many people would die of other causes before they ever got Alzheimer's disease.

Every pharmaceutical company worth its salt is therefore working on how to slow the progression or delay the first symptoms of

Alzheimer's disease. In general they are working in several basic areas. The first approach is to prevent the accumulation of the abnormal form of amyloid protein. The plaques that build up in the brains of people with Alzheimer's disease consist of fragments of amyloid protein. These fragments, called Aβ or A-beta, vary in length, but one particular length is especially toxic to nerve cells. Researchers are concentrating on either preventing this toxic fragment from accumulating or removing it from the brain. Genetically engineered "Alzheimer mice," who show the same toxic buildup in their brains as human patients do, are invaluable to this research.

Recently there have been two exciting developments. Scientists have discovered the crucial enzymes that allow the Aβ fragments to accumulate and have developed ways to modify these enzymes. When the enzymes are manipulated in the mouse models, plaques do not form in the animals' brains. Now the trick will be to develop drugs that will alter the enzymes safely in people. The race is on as we write. The statins, mentioned earlier, are another exciting development. It is not clear why they may delay the appearance of Alzheimer's disease. One possibility is that they lower cholesterol, thereby making it less likely that vascular disease of the brain is aggravating the Alzheimer's disease. An alternative explanation, however, is that the statins make it less easy for amyloid and its fragments to accumulate. This possibility has become a very hot area of research.

The second approach involves getting the body to use its immune system to remove the amyloid from the brain. A person is injected, that is, immunized, with the offending fragment of amyloid, and then makes antibodies to this fragment. The person's own antibodies attack and remove the amyloid. In the Alzheimer mice, the antibodies not only removed the amyloid plaques, they kept them from forming. Heavily diseased mice returned to normal. Clinical trials of this immunological approach in patients with Alzheimer's disease are in progress.

A third approach is to try to keep alive the nerve cells in which amyoloid is already accumulating. Two agents are currently being studied: vitamin E and estrogen. Substances called trophic factors also may help sustain these endangered cells. The brain normally deploys trophic factors in very small quantities to maintain the health of nerve cells. With the techniques of molecular biology, researchers can now make large amounts of these substances and try them out as drugs for treatment. The problem is getting trophic factors into the areas of the brain affected by the disease. One approach is to use genetic engineering—to put the gene that directs the production of the trophic factor into a bacterium that's been rendered harmless, then put the bacterium into the brain to deliver the gene to the brain cells. This sounds like science fiction but actually works in experimental animals. Preliminary trials of this gene therapy are under way in people.

The final strategy is to decrease the inflammation in the brain that occurs in response to the abnormal amyloid's attack on nerve cells. This approach takes its cue from recent advances in treating arthritis' inflammation in the joints with anti-inflammatory medications like aspirin, Motrin, or the recently FDA-approved COX-2 inhibitors. Studies are ongoing to see if these anti-inflammatory drugs have a role in treating Alzheimer's disease.

Only a few years ago medicine had no way to treat Alzheimer's disease. Now multiple avenues are under investigation. Some depend on the latest genetic and molecular engineering techniques, such as the mice that incorporate Alzheimer genes and the methods used to develop a vaccine to remove amyloid plaques. A century of study of patients with Alzheimer's disease finally shows signs of paying off. We feel that a new wave of treatments will become available in the near future.

FRONTOTEMPORAL DEMENTIA

After physicians realized that Alzheimer's disease was common in older as well as younger people, they then tended to think that almost all individuals with dementia had Alzheimer's disease. Now physicians recognize that other, rarer forms of dementia exist and that they require distinctive treatments of their own. Frontotemporal dementia is one of these disorders.

About the same time that Alois Alzheimer first described the disease bearing his name, another German physician, Arnold Pick, described a man in whom the very front of the brain—part of the frontal lobes, and the front parts of the temporal lobes—were dramatically shrunken, while the rest of brain appeared essentially normal. It was as if someone were separating the involved parts of the brain from the normal parts with a knife. In some patients the brain changes are more subtle, even though the symptoms are similar.

As many as 25 percent of patients who ultimately are diagnosed with frontotemporal dementia are misdiagnosed with Alzheimer's disease. But this form of dementia differs from Alzheimer's in several ways. First, in the majority of these patients the condition begins with behavior problems. Second, these symptoms most commonly begin when people are in their 50s and 60s and are quite uncommon among people who are very elderly—the reverse of Alzheimer's disease. Third, as we mentioned above, the anatomical changes in the brain that cause frontotemporal dementia are completely different from those seen in Alzheimer's disease. Finally, they have different genetic mechanisms. Instead of accumulating amyloid protein, the brains of some patients with frontotemporal dementia show a buildup of the protein, tau, the protein involved with the Alzheimer tangles. Close observations of behavior combined with an imaging test can make the distinction.

The Early Phase of Frontotemporal Dementia

The most common early symptom in frontotemporal dementia is a change in personality and behavior. A person starts doing things that are very uncharacteristic, often things that are very unusual by any standards. A person who is usually law abiding may begin shoplifting, or have an automobile accident and drive away unconcerned. Someone who is usually conservative and proper may start to swear, make improper advances to the opposite sex, buy seductive clothing and wear it in inappropriate places, or bet money indiscriminately. A person who is usually calm may become very irritable, a person who is a worrier may become exceedingly apathetic. Some people, of course, behave like this throughout their lives; the first sign of possible frontotemporal dementia is when these behaviors show up with increasing frequency as a dramatic change.

Harry was a 55-year-old banker who had been assigned to London by an American bank. He was quite successful primarily because he was a good "people person," and he adapted well to the new environment. The first indication that something was wrong surfaced in his interpersonal relationships at work. He became very short tempered, made erratic decisions, and began swearing at inappropriate times. Shortly thereafter, he became increasingly impulsive in his handling of money. It reached the point where his wife hid his credit cards to keep him from immediately responding to every TV advertisement for exercise machines or record collections. Harry had been very popular with his colleagues; initially they attempted to cover up for his altered behavior at work. However, they became concerned when one day he attempted to invest a lot of the bank's money in a high-risk venture without consulting anyone. When confronted, he seemed blasé. This convinced his colleagues that something was seriously wrong. They encouraged his wife to have him evaluated. Initially, physicians considered that he might be depressed and treated him on that basis without any effect. Further neurological evaluation, including careful neuropsychological testing and imaging of his brain, taken together with his medical history, ultimately led to the diagnosis of frontotemporal dementia.

It is naturally hard for friends or family members to accept that changes in a person's behavior are symptoms of a disease. Often it is not until people begin to have substantial problems with planning and organization that others realize that something is wrong and bring them in for evaluation. Eventually, problems spread to other areas of mental ability, such as memory.

In addition to causing changes in behavior, frontotemporal dementia can also begin with a language problem. This set of symptoms is very much like the unusual "language presentation" of Alzheimer's disease. Such individuals generally begin by having trouble finding the words to say what they want to say, at a time when they can still understand very well. Eventually, the person develops trouble reading, writing, and understanding what other people are saying. One symptom that can occur is "word deafness," a term which describes a person who, although still quite mildly impaired in other areas, can hear and repeat words clearly but be unable to understand them. For example, they may say, "window, what is a window?" Over time, other symptoms besides language difficulty begin to appear.

Alice, a very active 58-year-old member of her community, began having trouble speaking. At first, she would say the wrong word, or only parts of a word. Her family began to joke with her about how she was thinking faster than she was speaking. Over time, she spoke less and less. She could understand everything that people were saying to her and she could still read, but she ceased writing letters to friends. About 18 months after all this started, she did not speak at all except to make single unintelligible sounds. In a restaurant, she would point at the dishes she wanted in the menu, but could not say them. Because of her problems speaking, it was difficult to tell how much her language comprehension was affected. But she remembered friends and responded correctly, using hand signals to answer questions about news events that had been reported on television.

At about this time, her behavior began to change. She became very impulsive. She grabbed food off others' plates. She began losing things and suspected that people were stealing from her. When her husband hired household help, she accused them of stealing and insisted they be fired. She also developed certain obsessional characteristics. Things had to be in exactly the same place on the tables in the living room. She insisted on walking the same path every day; she began to sit reading the same book over and over for much of the day and got very upset if someone tried to give her a different book. It became very difficult for her husband to take her for a drive, because when they stopped (as for a red light), she got out of the car for no reason. It then became very difficult to persuade her to get back in the car again.

Alice's husband used behavioral management to reduce problems in daily life. He constantly reassured her that he loved her and that financial affairs were being taken care of, because he knew she worried about them. Because she could still understand everything that was going on, he periodically arranged for a small number of old friends to come for a drink or for dinner, and made sure to include her in the conversation. When Alice began to insist on doing the same things over and over again, he capitalized on this by arranging for her to walk to a neighbor's pool, where she swam long distances every day.

Treatment of Frontotemporal Dementia

Attempts to treat frontotemporal dementia have not been successful. Drugs like Aricept do not help. Mild sedation may help the behavior, but no ways to alter the course of the disease have been found.

Now that frontotemporal dementia has been recognized as a distinct disease, the progress in understanding and treating it is following the course that occurred with Alzheimer's disease. As in Alzheimer's disease, an abnormal protein, called tau, accumulates in the brains of some patients with the disease. Researchers have identified several families with genetic abnormalities in the processing of tau; strains of mice bred to have the same abnormality are being used to develop treatments. Progress should develop as rapidly as it has with Alzheimer's disease.

CREUTZFELD-JACOB DISEASE AND MAD COW DISEASE

Mary was less than four feet tall as a teenager. Starting at age 14, she received injections of human growth hormone over a period of seven to eight years. The preparation of growth hormone was made from pooled samples of human pituitary glands obtained from brains during autopsies.

Twenty years later, she began to be quite clumsy. While hiking with her husband, she could not walk along a narrow trail. Shortly thereafter trouble set in at work. As the office manager for a bank, she prided herself on her ability to remember the details of accounts. Within a few months she couldn't remember crucial details that previously were second nature to her. Her boss made her the receptionist, but soon even those duties were too much for her.

Her coordination and memory functions deteriorated very rapidly, and she died eight months after the start of her symptoms. When her brain was examined, it was found that she had Creutzfeld-Jacob Disease (CJD), a progressive degeneration of the brain. Impossible as it sounds, she contracted the disease from the growth hormone she received as a teenager.

CJD is a currently untreatable form of dementia, and fortunately it is quite rare, affecting only one person in a million worldwide; in the United States there are about 200 cases per year. CJD is a rapidly progressing dementia. Because the typical age of onset is around 60, and the symptoms include memory loss, behavioral changes, and lack of coordination, the condition is often mistaken for Alzheimer's disease or some other neurological disorder. A physician cannot check for Creutzfeld-Jacob Disease with a simple blood or urine test. Diagnosis requires examining the brain tissue. Since the implications of CJD are so serious—the disease is fatal virtually 100 percent of the time—physicians often obtain a small sample of brain tissue through a tiny hole in the skull to confirm the diagnosis.

CJD appears "out of the blue." No symptoms appear beforehand to give warning. The disease is not easy to catch. It can't be transmitted through the air or through casual contact, and spouses and family members are not at increased risk of contracting it. In unusual situations CJD is spread through direct contact with infected brain tissue. For example, neurosurgeons have contracted CJD after operating on a patient with it. Similarly, a cornea transplant can carry the disease from the donor to the recipient (CJD also attacks eye tissue). Contracting the disease from injections with growth hormone, as Mary did, is no longer a danger. Since 1985, all human growth hormone used in the United States has been synthesized using sophisticated DNA techniques, thus eliminating the chance of infection through that route.

Although the chances of contracting CJD are extremely slight, fears about a related condition, Mad Cow Disease, are on the rise due to a well-publicized outbreak in 1985 in England. The diseases have a unique mechanism. Instead of resulting from infection by bacteria or viruses, CJD and its animal-infecting counterparts are diseases in which a group of proteins called prions, which are normally present in the brain, develop abnormal structures consisting of strange folds. When these misfolded proteins come in contact with normal prions they induce the normal proteins to assume abnormal shapes. Ultimately, enough abnormal prions accumulate to start to kill nerve cells.

The 1985 outbreak of Mad Cow Disease started in a group of calves whose feed contained "renderings"—ground up meat and bone meal—from sheep infected with another prion disease, called scrapie. The renderings were produced under a new system that did not kill the scrapie agent, thus infecting the cows. The British government killed thousands of older animals, in case they harbored the disease, and the practice of feeding animals with sheep renderings prepared in this manner has stopped. The result is that the disease in cattle has markedly disappeared in Great Britain, but it has appeared in France and Germany.

In the last few years, about 100 people in England have developed a prion disease. The disease, called CJ variant, is a little different from the form that Mary had. These victims are younger; they first have behavioral problems and then go on to develop clumsiness and dementia. Analysis of the brains of patients who die from the disease shows the same abnormally folded prions as in cows with Mad Cow Disease. Concern abounds that these people got the disease from eating British beef.

Scientists are watching very carefully to see if there is any evidence of increased numbers of CJ variant disease in England. One problem is that due to the lack of a definitive diagnostic test for either cattle or people, no one knows how many people in Britain might be harboring the disease. Precautions are being taken, however. To prevent any possibility of the disease being spread by blood transfusion;

Americans who lived in England during the 1980s and might have been exposed to British beef are not allowed to donate blood in the United States.

CJD and Mad Cow Disease remain mysteries. Even when a person is exposed to the abnormal prion protein there is a very long interval before they develop the disorder. Mary's story demonstrates how long the interval between exposure to the agent and the onset of the disease can be. It is not entirely clear what is going on in the brain during this long silent phase of the disorder. Medical science badly needs a test that can determine whether a person has been exposed to abnormal prions and is in the process of developing the disease. Once a reliable test is developed, drugs to treat the disease may come from several chemical agents that can keep proteins from folding in abnormal ways.

Despite the fact that Mad Cow Disease has affected thousands of sheep and cows, there have been only 100 human cases, with no increasing frequency. Dire predictions of a human epidemic, possibly involving thousands of people, have not come true. European health authorities have devised new regulations to identify the disease in cattle and have banned the feeding practices that led to the contamination. With each passing year, the chances of your getting CJD are less and less likely, even if you ate British beef in the late 1980s and 1990s.

WHAT YOU CAN DO ABOUT ALZHEIMER'S DISEASE AND OTHER DEMENTIAS: RESOURCES AND OPTIONS FOR CAREGIVERS

Alzheimer's disease can be a frighteningly complicated problem to handle. To reduce the burden as much as possible, take advantage of any and all available help. The first step is to be well informed. The Alzheimer's Association, the primary advocacy group within the United States, acts as a clearinghouse for comprehensive and reliable information (see the Appendix at the back of this book). Many excellent books are in print to help families and caregivers get a handle on this terrible disease; for example, one called *The 36-Hour Day: A Family Guide to Caring for Persons with Alzheimer's Disease, Related Dementing Illnesses, and Memory Loss in Later Life,* by Nancy L. Mace and Peter V. Rabins, has sold nearly a quarter of a million copies.

If nursing home care is not a possibility, keep in mind that there are other options. Around larger metropolitan areas, Alzheimer's families can work with their doctors to use the guidance and counseling services in the many hospital complexes that have Alzheimer's centers and clinics. Counselors in these services can help determine eligibility for entitlement or visiting home health care workers. They can also steer you towards programs including:

- *Adult day care,* which may include small group and individual activities; nutritious meals; transportation; nursing care; family counseling; and occupational, speech, and physical therapies.
- *Respite care,* designed precisely to give caregivers a much-needed break. Respite care includes adult day care and home care services, as well as overnight stays in a facility, and can be provided a few hours a week or for a weekend. For many families, respite care mean the difference between keeping patients at home and placing them in an institution before they really need to be there.
- *Home care,* which combines health care and supportive services to let homebound or disabled persons continue their accustomed way of life as much as possible. Home care can consist of visits by a volunteer from a community service or religious group; a health aide to help for a few hours a day or week to assist in household duties or personal care (bathing, dressing, shopping, and cleaning); or a nurse or other health professional to assist with medical as well as personal care. The expense rises with the level of expertise. Medicare, Medicaid, and some insurance policies pay for limited home care.

Families who can afford care outside of the home have several options, ranging from assisted living and residential care facilities—good for those who can live somewhat independently and have no serious medical needs—or skilled nursing or special needs facilities. Anyone making this often heartbreaking decision will want to make sure the home is a good one. When choosing a facility, keep in mind:

- A number of publications are available that provide checklists to help families and caregivers evaluate the physical environment, staffing patterns, activities, and services. These include inspection of safety procedures, visiting policies, cleanliness, attentiveness of nursing staff, quality of food, and availability of pharmaceuticals and laundry services. (For these publications contact the advocacy groups; see Appendix.)
- Lists of facilities, background information, advocacy, and investigation of problems are available from local ombudsman offices statewide and across the country. Help in finding a facility also may be available from a hospital discharge planner or social worker.

Though costs can be staggering, some help is available, depending on the person's economic circumstances and the level of care required. The primary financing option for most individuals in skilled nursing homes, as well as some rehabilitation facilities, is the Medicaid program (Medi-Cal in California). Medicaid will only pay for care that is deemed medically necessary. For this, families must meet income eligibility requirements and may have to "spend down" their assets in accordance with federal and state guidelines to qualify for this public benefit. Provisions are also available to protect the assets of the well spouse. For those not eligible, some loans are available, such a reverse annuity mortgage, which converts home equity into a monthly cash stipend to pay for long-term care. Consult with an attorney who specializes in estate planning and public benefits, and check all lenders with the Better Business Bureau or other local consumer groups.

CHAPTER 15

TREATABLE DEMENTIAS

Dementia is a loss of mental ability that can impair a person's ability to function. Though the word makes many people immediately think of Alzheimer's disease, some forms of dementia can be treated, making it extremely important to identify them accurately. The causes of dementia include unusual infections and various illnesses related to the chemistry of the body—all of which could affect young people, even children, as well. In the elderly, however, these conditions can cloud diagnosis; their symptoms overlap with those of less treatable disorders such as Alzheimer's disease. Some of these disorders require surgery; others respond well to medicines alone.

SUBDURAL HEMATOMA

Helen, a prominent Washington lawyer, aged 58, began having episodes of confusion and loss of memory. The people in her law firm chose to ignore the early signs of trouble, perhaps to avoid embarrassing her. The problem became more complicated when it turned out that she was drinking to excess at night and on weekends. Several physicians saw her but attributed her problems to alcohol and did not look for an underlying cause. Eventually her performance at work became so erratic that an old friend and fellow lawyer stepped in and insisted that she be reevaluated.

On examination, she looked well and was not sure why she was seeing her doctor. From her medical history, the physician learned that several years ago she had suffered a heart attack and since then had been taking blood thinners. She could not recall any falls or head injury. She was very confused, not knowing the date other than the year, and not knowing what hospital she was in. As a test, the doctor showed her three objects and asked her to remember them; afterward, she could not do so. Other aspects of her memory were equally impaired. The only clue to her problem was that she didn't move the right side of her face as much as the left when she smiled or talked.

An MRI revealed that her brain was being distorted by not one but two collections of blood between the inside of her skull and the surface of her brain. The neurosurgeon removed these collections. It took about a week before she began to recover, but by a month after the surgery, she was back to her normal self. Only then was she able to remember that she had hit her head about a month before. While playing golf, she was riding in her golf cart and bumped her head on the branch of a tree. Because of her blood thinners, that slight bump was enough to start some bleeding in the subdural space between her skull and brain.

Helen's story illustrates the typical progress of dementia resulting from a subdural hematoma. The process is sneaky. A person may not remember the head injury, often quite minor, that started the problem. The progression of the decline in memory and other thinking processes can be very gradual. Recognition is crucial because the condition is quite treatable.

What Is the Cause of Subdural Hematoma?

The skull is a closed box with a finite amount of space that is taken up by the brain, blood vessels, and fluid that washes over them (called cerebrospinal fluid). If something else occupies part of that space, then pressure inside the skull increases and the brain gets squeezed. When that happens, the brain does not work normally, and thinking and memory can decline. A subdural hematoma occurs when a collection of blood between the brain and the skull presses on the brain. Ultimately the pressure from this blood will alter mental ability.

Treatment of Subdural Hematoma

During the early stages of dementia, imaging studies such as CT and MRI can catch treatable conditions before they do irreversible damage. For example, they can help diagnose a subdural hematoma by revealing a collection of blood on the outside of the brain. Treatment usually involves drilling a small hole in the skull and removing the blood. This procedure is risky, however, and it isn't always necessary. Some hematomas are absorbed by the brain; it is a good idea to repeat the imaging studies to see if this is the case.

The future may bring refinements to present techniques, but the important thing is to use the ones already available. The advent of rapid, noninvasive imaging of the brain, such as CT and MRI, represents a huge advance in diagnosing and managing subdural hematomas. If there is one test that every person with progressive memory loss should have, it is proper imaging to rule out this diagnosis.

Hydrocephalus ("Water on the Brain")

Marty, a 74-year-old retired insurance agent, felt unsteady on his feet when he went out in the morning to pick up his newspaper at the end of the driveway. One morning he fell while bending over and had difficulty getting back up and into the house. About the same time, he began having trouble controlling his bladder. On two occasions he wet his bed. He was very embarrassed by this problem and did not tell his wife or children. What brought him to medical attention was that he could no longer keep track of things. He forgot to balance his checkbook, failed to cash his Social Security check, and did not enter his financial data into a computer system he had used for the last few years—all of which was very unusual behavior for him.

On examination, he walked in a strange way, with his feet wide apart. He had difficulty turning and shuffled his feet, almost as if they were stuck to the floor. His memory was quite poor for a man of his age and educational background. On an MRI of his brain the spaces that contain fluid, called the ventricles, were much too big. Other tests measured the pressure inside his head and found that it was too high.

Marty had hydrocephalus (also known as water on the brain), a condition in which excess fluid builds up in the brain and causes pressure. He underwent surgery, during which a tube called a shunt was placed in his brain to drain off the excess fluid. All three of his symptoms—the problem with walking and balance, the incontinence, and the memory problems—abated and he soon recovered completely.

About two years later, we got a call from Marty's wife. Every Sunday, Marty used to bring her coffee in bed. This required that he climb the stairs carrying the coffee. Gradually he was having trouble balancing the coffee and was spilling more and more. Marty's wife was concerned that his shunt might have stopped working. She was right. A part of it had become plugged up, and was fixed with a simple operation. Now he is back to normal again. And his wife has invented a new way of following how Marty is doing—the "coffee-carrying index."

What Causes Hydrocephalus?

The human brain produces about one or two cups of cerebrospinal fluid each day. This fluid flows from deep inside the brain, circulates around the brain tissue and spinal cord, and is then reabsorbed, by a process that is very much like a circulating pump in a fountain. Sometimes this fluid is not reabsorbed the way it should be, and begins to build up inside the brain. This may occur because of a blow to the head, but occasionally there is no particular cause that anyone can point to. When the fluid starts to accumulate, and the channels within the brain through which fluid flows expand, then hydrocephalus is produced.

Treatment of Hydrocephalus

Like subdural hematomas, the diagnosis of hydrocephalus is often overlooked. Proper imaging of the brain is essential to identify this condition. The treatment involves placing a tube in the brain and draining out the fluid that is accumulating. This tube acts as a shunt, giving the fluid an escape route. The tube runs from the spaces in the brain that contain the largest amount of fluid (the ventricles), out through a small hole in the skull, under the skin, and down into the abdomen, where the fluid can be absorbed.

Before such a procedure is performed, the neurologist measures the pressure in the brain to see if it is abnormal. This is done through a spinal tap, in which a small needle is placed in the back to check the pressure in the cerebrospinal fluid. If the pressure is too high, then an operation is recommended. Occasionally, continuous monitoring of the pressure is necessary to determine if the pressure has increased. One of the ways to determine if a shunt will be successful is to remove a small amount of cerebrospinal fluid, and then follow the patient's symptoms to see if they improve. If they do, then it is likely that the shunt will help, and surgery is recommended.

If the shunt is successful in relieving symptoms, it must be worn for the rest of a person's life. This creates an ongoing risk of an infection. The body does not like to have foreign objects like shunt tubes in place for long periods of time, and they can easily become infected. When that happens, the shunt tube must be removed and person treated with antibiotics. A new shunt can then be inserted. The second problem, as occurred with Marty, is that the shunt tube can become clogged and stop working. Sometimes it is possible to unplug the shunt. More commonly, the shunt has to be replaced.

Future Treatments of Hydrocephalus

For some patients, as for Marty, placing a shunt to relieve hydrocephalus can be spectacularly successful. However, it is difficult to predict ahead of time if a shunting procedure will actually help. Part of the problem is that individuals with diseases involving memory loss or difficulty walking, such as Alzheimer's disease and Parkinson's disease, can also have enlarged ventricles. The challenge is how to determine who will benefit from treatment. Researchers are devising new methods to monitor the pressure inside the brain to determine if the shunt should be installed. These techniques may also be used to see if the shunt is having a beneficial effect.

PROBLEMS THINKING AND BLOOD VESSEL DISEASE

Angelo, a 72-year-old shopkeeper, had a history of multiple medical problems including high blood pressure, diabetes, and a heart attack when he was 64. Nevertheless, he continued to operate his grocery store six days a week. On Sundays, with help from his wife, Maria, he figured out what to order during the coming week. Maria noticed that Angelo was repeating the same orders every week, making no allowance for the changing seasons of the year. He also became more irritable, arguing with the delivery people and being much less tolerant of the children who came into the store. This irritability was particularly striking because Angelo was widely liked and had always had a fondness for children. One morning, while standing at his cash register, Angelo had trouble using his left hand for a few minutes. This scared him, and he went to his physician.

Because he had so many illnesses that suggested disease of the blood vessels, his physician had an MRI done. This revealed numerous small abnormalities in his brain, indicating many small areas of vascular damage. As a result, Angelo's physician decided to use stronger medication to keep his blood pressure under control. He also emphasized how important it was for Angelo to follow his treatment routines by taking his medicine on schedule, monitoring his diabetes and blood pressure, and taking aspirin each day. Fortunately, Maria had accompanied Angelo on his medical visit, and she also heard the doctor's warnings. Between the two of them, Angelo changed his ways.

Over the next few months, Angelo did not get strikingly better. However, his symptoms, which had been getting progressively worse, leveled off. He is still running the grocery, but he has brought in someone to help him with the ordering and bookkeeping.

Angelo is a good example of what can happen when the small vessels of the brain are damaged by long-standing illnesses, such as diabetes and hypertension. The damage is not confined to a single large area of the brain, as occurs with a stroke, but rather extends to multiple small areas throughout the brain. The symptoms depend on what parts of the brain are involved. It is common for patients to have trouble with planning and with handling complex ideas, to be unable to control their emotions, and to have a general slowness of movement. Memory is sometimes affected, but is usually not the primary problem. Angelo's problem is often called "vascular dementia."

What Causes Vascular Dementia?

High blood pressure, diabetes, high cholesterol, and smoking, among other things, can gradually lead to the narrowing of small blood vessels, and this in turn can cause problems with thinking. If this is the case, an MRI will show numerous small areas of damage, reflecting the fact that small blood vessels are not delivering enough blood to these regions of the brain. Dozens of small abnormalities may be visible; many more may be too small to see.

Treatments of Vascular Dementia

When a person with problems thinking has a history of high blood pressure and/or diabetes, and an MRI shows damage from the narrowing of small blood vessels, treatment should focus on preventing additional damage to blood vessels in the brain. The first line of defense is to control the underlying diseases. That means to be sure that conditions such as high blood pressure, diabetes, or high cholesterol are addressed, and that the patient change bad lifestyle habits such as smoking.

Many physicians also treat vascular dementia with aspirin or other compounds that keep blood from clotting. Although commonly used, there is no clear-cut evidence that they actually make a difference. The whole area of vascular dementia is confused by differing criteria for diagnosis and very few long-term studies. Nevertheless, we use aspirin for these patients.

Part of the damage in blood vessel disease represents inflammation of the brain tissue, which appears to be part of the immune system's response to the damaged tissue. As is also the case in stroke and Alzheimer's disease, the body's immune response compounds the problem instead of eliminating it. Thus, one of the newer approaches to treatment is to use anti-inflammatory drugs such as ibuprofen or medicines known as COX-2 inhibitors. Studies to see if such medications will be more effective than aspirin alone are under way.

LYME DISEASE

Michael and his brother were builders on Block Island, an island off the coast of Long Island in New York. Michael was outside a lot because of his work, and he also enjoyed going for long walks in the woods around the island. He began to experience headaches, which were unusual for him, and aches in his joints. He treated these symptoms with ibuprofen and went on working. Michael normally handled the books of his business on Sundays. He noticed he was making mistakes; he couldn't remember what he had ordered and used during the previous week. His brother, who often helped him with the bookkeeping, noticed that the bills were not going out as they should, and took over those duties.

Michael finally went to see his physician. She asked him if he had noticed a rash at about the time that he started feeling achy. He thought he had, but wasn't very sure. Since Block Island is a hotbed of Lyme disease, she immediately sent off a blood test. The results were inconclusive. Still uncertain, she obtained some cerebrospinal fluid by a lumbar puncture and sent it to a special laboratory, which runs more specific tests for Lyme disease. While waiting for the results, she decided to treat Michael as if he had the disease, using an antibiotic called Doxycycline. Two or three weeks later, the special tests came back positive, establishing the diagnosis. In the meantime, Michael's symptoms had already begun to improve. Now certain of the diagnosis, Michael's physician treated him even more vigorously, using antibiotics given intravenously. It took several months for Michael to feel that he was totally back to normal.

Lyme disease is a relatively new illness that was first described in the United States in the 1970s. In the beginning, it was thought to only cause arthritis in children, but we now know that it affects people of all ages and often involves the brain. In older people the disease can be confused with other conditions, such as arthritis and forms of memory impairment such as Alzheimer's disease. Symptoms can be varied. At the start of the infection, they can include skin rash, headaches, pain in the arms and legs, and an inability to move the muscles of the face. Later in the course of the disease, months or even years after the initial infection, symptoms such as memory loss and numbness in the hands and the feet can occur.

The symptoms of the early phase of the disease can be very distinctive, such as a rash that looks like a gradually expanding bull's-eye around the area of a tick bite. Other symptoms of the early phase include headache, fever, trouble thinking, and pains in the arms and feet. When a person who has been in a region with a lot of Lyme Disease has these symptoms, we assume it is Lyme disease until proven otherwise.

The symptoms of the late phase, however, are often confusing and difficult to diagnose. Some people either did not have, or do not remember having, the skin rash and do not have any of the other symptoms often seen in the early phase. Nevertheless, over a period of weeks or months, they develop problems with memory or depression. They may also have trouble walking and feeling things with their feet and hands.

What Causes Lyme Disease?

Lyme disease is caused by an organism, called a spirochete, and is spread by ticks that pick up this organism by biting infected mice and deer. Typically, Lyme disease develops in people who are outside, walking in the woods and high grass. Some people can get Lyme disease without going into the woods; cats and dogs can carry an infected tick into the house, where it can jump from the pet to the person.

Treatment of Lyme Disease

To diagnose Lyme disease physicians employ a blood test that detects antibodies to the spirochete. Although widely used, the test is imperfect. It can be negative if it is given too soon and the antibodies have not had time to develop. In addition, the test will be positive in people who have received the vaccine for Lyme disease. Special laboratories can perform additional tests to establish the diagnosis, as was done for Michael.

In the early phase of Lyme disease, patients take an antibiotic known as Doxycycline. In the later phase, they may require a stronger antibiotic, such as Ceftriaxone, given intravenously for at least three weeks. The sooner treatment with antibiotics begins, the more quickly a person will recover.

The problems in both diagnosis and treatment center around people who have late manifestations, or chronic Lyme disease. Some clearly had established acute Lyme disease, were treated with antibiotics, but still had symptoms. Others never clearly had Lyme disease. Both groups often have symptoms of depression, problems with memory, fatigue, and may have abnormal feelings in their hands and feet. A recent study compared using high dosages of antibiotics versus no treatment and found no differences in outcome. So, at present it is not clear what is actually wrong with these people, nor are we certain how to treat them.

In the United States, a vaccine called Lymerix has been developed. It requires three doses, given over a one-year period. In the first year, a person has only about half the protection the vaccine eventually provide. After the three treatments are complete, the vaccine is 70 to 80 percent effective.

The best way to treat Lyme disease is not to get it in the first place. When walking in the woods, wear long-sleeved shirts and tuck your pants legs into your socks. Remember that ordinary dog ticks don't cause the disease; the culprits are pinhead-sized. Light-colored clothing will make ticks more visible. To cause Lyme disease the tick needs to be attached and sucking blood for at least 24 hours, so check yourself and your pets carefully every time you come in. When removing the ticks, don't try to crush them with your fingers.

In the short period of time since Lyme disease emerged, research has identified the infectious agent and developed both diagnostic tests and a vaccine. However, physicians and patients still need better diagnostic tests and more effective treatments, as Michael's case shows. A more reliable vaccine is also needed. With better vaccines, Lyme disease could follow other similar disorders, such as polio and smallpox, into oblivion.

WHAT YOU CAN DO ABOUT TREATABLE DEMENTIAS: THE IMPORTANCE OF QUICK DIAGNOSIS

Treatable dementias are instances where medical consultation is the primary action a person needs to take. Each cause and treatment will be specific for the individual and it's important to carefully follow the physician's advice after treatment has started. In many cases, especially when the condition and its treatment continue for a long time, an organization exists that provides information and services for backup information and assistance (see the Appendix in the back of this book). Too often, the person or others who notice the symptoms of treatable dementias will put them together with the person's age and jump to the conclusion that it might be Alzheimer's, which usually means they'll decide to wait and see instead of saying anything. That is how bad mistakes are made.

CHAPTER 16

CANCER AND THE BRAIN

In 1945, Marilyn was talking to her grandmother Rose when Rose had an epileptic seizure for the first time in her life at age 62. After the seizure cleared, Rose had some trouble talking and using her right hand. Everyone assumed that she had had a stroke. This was, of course, long before current imaging techniques such as CT and MRI scanning had been developed. There were only two ways to get an idea of what was going on in her brain: to introduce air to outline the brain (a procedure known as pneumoencephalography, which is not done anymore), or to outline the arteries of the brain with a dye (a procedure called an arteriogram, which was just being developed). Neither of these procedures was done initially on Rose because they could produce serious side effects and, if she had had a stroke, might have caused more problems than they solved.

Over the next month, however, her speaking problems became worse and she could no longer walk or use her right hand. This pattern of progressive difficulty did not follow the normal course after a stroke. Eventually Rose's doctors performed a pneumonoencephalogram, which revealed an enormous abnormal growth, about the size of an orange, pressing on the left side of her brain. In a surgical procedure that took over 16 hours, this growth was completely removed.

Within two weeks, Rose was up walking and starting to talk again. After months of rehabilitation, the only permanent problem she had from the surgery was difficulty with the fine motor coordination of her right hand. She could still knit but she could not sew, and her handwriting was quite poor because she had trouble holding a pen or pencil. The tumor never recurred during the next 37 years of her life.

Tumors begin when the "brakes" on cell growth give out and cells begin to divide uncontrollably. Brain tumors can involve just the covering of the brain, as with Rose, or they can involve the substance of the brain itself. Alternatively, they can spread to the brain from other organs, such as the lung or breast, causing what we call a metastatic brain tumor.

Cancer can also affect the brain indirectly. The body's reaction to cancer in some other organ may produce changes in the immune system that harm the brain, for example, impairing functions such as mental ability or control of coordination. In addition, many treatments that are used for all forms of cancer have side effects that can produce problems with brain and nerve functions.

WHAT ARE THE SYMPTOMS OF BRAIN TUMORS?

Certain types of complaints or changes lead a doctor to suspect that an older person might have some form of brain tumor. These include headache in someone who normally does not get them, an epileptic seizure, a change in personality, or difficulty moving correctly.

Headaches

Headaches are extremely common. Some people have them all their lives, but those aren't the people whose headaches cause concern. The people who need attention are those who almost never had headaches before and suddenly start complaining of them. Brain tumors cause pain because the skull is like a closed box with a finite amount of room inside. When a tumor starts growing and taking up space, the components of the brain have to shift to make room for the tumor; as the tumor gets larger, the pressure inside the skull also increases. Both of these reactions to the tumor cause headaches.

Seizures

When an older person has a seizure for the first time, there is almost always a discernible cause. Sometimes the seizure is triggered by a stroke or a head injury, and sometimes, as with Rose, it indicates a brain tumor. The seizure offers no clues as to the type of tumor, but it suggests that a tumor is present.

Behavioral Changes

Problems with memory, apathy, loss of initiative, or other changes in personality can be early warning signs of a number of brain disorders, such as Alzheimer's disease or depression. They can also be related to a brain tumor, usually in the front part of the brain. The cause of these behavioral symptoms can be hard to sort out on clinical examination, which is one reason why people with possible dementia undergo brain imaging studies as part of their evaluation. Dementing disorders such as Alzheimer's disease cannot yet be cured, but it is often possible to find and remove a tumor if that is the real culprit.

Language and Motor Symptoms

The symptoms of a brain tumor depend on where the tumor is. If it is in a part of the brain associated with language, or in the part associated with movement, the enlarging tumor will disrupt these parts of the brain and cause the specific problems in language or movement, like those that affected Rose.

HOW IS A BRAIN TUMOR DIAGNOSED?

If a doctor suspects a brain tumor, the first step is to do an imaging study of the brain. An MRI is the best choice; a CT scan is slightly less accurate because some parts of the brain are hard to see with that technique. The MRI shows whether or not there is a tumor, but usually not what type. To determine that, a piece of the tumor must be removed by a procedure called a biopsy, and examined under the microscope. The biopsy involves making a tiny hole in the skull and removing a piece of the tumor with a small probe. To position the instrument correctly, the surgeon looks at a picture of the brain with an MRI machine. This way, the surgeon can see exactly where the probe is, and can take small selective samples with little or no damage to the normal surrounding structures. The patient often goes home the next day.

The piece of the tumor is then examined under the microscope, sometimes using special stains to characterize the cells of the tumor. The first question to be answered is whether the problem is a tumor, or is it something else? Sometimes we get fooled, and what looked like a tumor turns out to be some form of infection—a much more treatable situation. Secondly, if it is a tumor, did it arise in the brain or come to the brain from some other tissue such as the breast or lung? Finally, if it is a primary brain tumor, how bad is it?

WHAT CAUSES BRAIN TUMORS?

No one knows what causes brain tumors. Scientists have tried to determine whether there are environmental or genetic factors that set the stage for brain cancer, but with very little success. The fastest-growing type of tumor occurs more commonly as people get older, so it appears that more women have this aggressive type of brain tumor, but that is because they live longer. People are always looking for potential environmental causes of brain tumors, but so far no one cause has been identified. For example, the increasing use of cell phones has evoked suspicions that they are responsible for a similar increase in the number of tumors known as glial tumors, but that speculation has not held up.

TUMORS ON THE OUTSIDE OF THE BRAIN

Marilyn's grandmother, Rose, had a brain tumor called a meningioma, caused by the slow growth of the cells that make up the coverings of the brain (the meninges). Because meningiomas grow so slowly, the brain initially can adjust to their increasing size. These tumors push brain structures out of the way gradually, so they can become very large before they are detected. Today's modern imaging procedures enable physicians to see and evaluate tumors like Rose's early on, rather than wait many weeks while they grow larger.

Until recently, surgeons removed meningiomas by opening the brain and taking them out. Now a new procedure using radiation, called a gamma knife, can dissolve the tumors without actual surgery. Meningiomas are totally curable. Sometimes they cannot be completely removed and grow back over many years, making it necessary to remove them again. However, they do not spread to the inside of the brain and they do not spread to other organs.

Tumors can also develop from the membranes that cover nerves. The most common of such tumors arise from the coverings of the nerve that carries signals for hearing, the acoustic nerve. Like meningiomas, acoustic nerve tumors grow very slowly. But they create their own unique symptoms. Because they press on the acoustic nerve, they disturb hearing, often producing a ringing sound and then eventually loss of hearing in one ear. A person may first notice a problem hearing the telephone in one ear. As the tumors enlarge, they affect other nearby nerves, particularly those that control the movements of one side of the face. These tumors can be seen by brain imaging, but sometimes it takes special scanning techniques to see them clearly. The surgery for these tumors is tricky, because the acoustic nerve passes by numerous vital brain structures. In expert hands, they are curable.

TUMORS ON THE INSIDE OF THE BRAIN

Jerry was a 65-year-old owner of a bookstore who was brought to the emergency room because he had just had a seizure. He had been standing at the counter talking to a customer when he suddenly stopped talking and seemed to stare off into space. Then his right arm and the right side of his face began to twitch, and he had difficulty talking. The customer called another salesperson in the store, who phoned for an ambulance. In the emergency room, Jerry was very confused and still had some difficulty talking. An MRI was immediately performed and showed a small tumor on the left side of his brain. The next day some of the tissue in the tumor was removed by a surgeon and examined immediately under a microscope. The tumor consisted of cells that looked relatively normal; there were just too many of them. This meant it was a slow-growing tumor, so the surgeon removed all that he could detect.

After the surgery, the area of the brain that had been occupied by the tumor was also exposed to radiation in order to kill any residual tumor cells. It has now been five years since the surgery and Jerry is doing very well. He is taking medication to prevent having any further seizures, and every year he has repeat imaging studies, which have not shown any return of the tumor.

Tumors inside the brain develop from cells of the brain, called glial cells. These are some of the so-called support cells, which do not transmit nerve impulses but carry out tasks essential to the brain's "housekeeping," like mopping up excess chemicals. Sometimes glial tumors grow very slowly and a person can live a normal life for many years before trouble occurs, as Jerry did. Other glial cell tumors grow very quickly and contain cells that divide very rapidly. Medicine does not yet have effective means for treating such fast growing tumors.

Looking at pieces of brain tissue under a microscope can determine a tumor's type. Physicians use a grading system of 1 to 4. A tumor in the grade 1 or 2 category, like Jerry's, is expected to be slow growing and may not even require any treatment at all, whereas those in grade 4 have a distinctive name (glioblastoma) and grow rapidly.

Glioblastomas are the ones that give brain tumors such a bad name. They are more common in the elderly and, despite current treatments, are often associated with a life expectancy of $\frac{1}{12}$–2 years after diagnosis. This is the type of brain tumor for which we desperately need new forms of treatment.

TUMORS THAT SPREAD TO THE BRAIN

A surgeon we know began having headaches. He had never had the problem before, but his wife had a long history of migraine, so he took some of her antiheadache medicine and went on working. One day while performing surgery, he looked up quickly and suddenly felt very unsteady on his feet. He was afraid he was going to fall. This feeling only lasted a few seconds, but it was enough for him to turn to his assistant and say, "Please finish this operation for me." He walked out of the operating room and called Guy and said, "I have a problem. I think I have a brain tumor." This is the kind of assumption Guy would have taken with a grain of salt had it come from anyone else.

When Guy examined him, there was clearly something the matter with his coordination, particularly in the use of his right hand, and he had difficulty when he tried to stand with his feet together. Guy immediately did an imaging study of his brain. The sugeon was right. There was a single small tumor in the back part of his brain, in the cerebellum, the part that influences balance. Otherwise he seemed quite healthy. He was not a smoker, he had not lost any weight, and he had no pain except for the recent headaches. X-rays of his lungs appeared normal. He had nothing to suggest he had cancer anywhere else.

The next day, the small tumor was removed from his brain. A study of the cells in the tumor, obtained by biopsy, indicated that they had originally come from his lung. Very careful x-rays were done again of his lungs, and a tiny cancerous growth was found which was removed through a small tube. He was given radiation to both his lungs and his brain, and a continuing course of chemotherapy. Four years later, he is doing very well. He has stopped performing surgery but he comes to the hospital every day to teach young doctors and medical students. He is also playing golf, which he always wanted more time to do. His major problem is with sensation in his feet, caused by the chemotherapy he was given. Because the chemotherapy can interfere with the normal signaling from nerves, the patient has a constant feeling of burning pain. He considers this a small price to pay for being alive and otherwise healthy.

Cancers can spread from one organ to another when little bits of tumor break off and enter the bloodstream. They then can be carried to other organs, where they set up shop. The cancers that spread to the brain most frequently are those common in the elderly: cancers of the lung, the breast, the bowel, and a cancer of the skin called malignant melanoma. Cancer of the prostate is a special case, because for some reason it spreads to the coverings of the brain rather than to the brain tissue itself.

When cancer spreads to the brain, it often grows as a single tumor. Thus, a metastatic brain tumor can have the same symptoms as a primary brain tumor and can look very much the same on an imaging study. Doctors can tell the difference only by looking at the tumor under a microscope and recognizing that the cells that make up the tumor do not normally exist in the brain, but have journeyed there from the lung or breast, for example. Sometimes, symptoms from the brain are the first sign that any form of cancer is present. At other times, the brain gets involved quite late in the disease, after the cancer has already spread to other organs.

TREATMENTS FOR BRAIN TUMORS

Treatment depends on the location and nature of the brain tumor. Some tumors like Rose's can be completely removed by surgery. In other cases, such as slow growing glial tumors or some cancers that have spread from other organs to the brain, surgical removal of the tumor may not be complete but can reduce the symptoms and considerably prolong quality of life, as it did for the surgeon who had lung cancer that spread to his brain.

The type of tumor that poses the biggest treatment problem is the bad form of glial tumor, the glioblastoma. This tumor usually spreads widely through the brain. Surgery can establish the diagnosis but cannot remove all of the tumor. After surgery, doctors use radiation and chemotherapy to try and kill the remaining cancer cells Currently these additional treatments are only partially successful.

Despite the disappointing results of efforts to treat most glioblastomas, the outlook for people with brain tumors has improved remarkably in recent years, particularly with respect to tumors that have spread from other organs (such as the breast or the lung). Previously if the brain became involved, medicine could do almost nothing. Now, as with the surgeon we described above, there are times when aggressive treatment, often a combination of surgery, radiation, and chemotherapy, can make a significant difference.

Research in Brain Tumors

The last few years have brought remarkable advances in the diagnosis and treatment of brain tumors, including newer forms of imaging for rapid diagnosis and surgery on the brain in combination with guidance from imaging (called stereotactic surgery). A breakthrough in removing tumors is the gamma knife, in which surgeons focus radiation very precisely at the tumor. This procedure is faster, safer, and much easier on an older person than the conventional operative approach.

Many researchers are trying to come up with better therapies for the worst tumor, the glioblastoma. One approach is to put cancer-fighting medications directly into the tumor in the form of a slow-release wafer. This approach extends both survival and quality of life, but so far has not produced cures. Modern genetic techniques are also being tried that can introduce genes into the tumor, in the hope that they will either kill the tumor or make it more responsive to treatment with chemotherapy or radiation. To aid this research, scientists are able to produce brain tumors in laboratory animals, and then are able to see how new ways of delivering chemicals to the brain or genetic treatments affect them. If the new techniques prove safe and effective, human trials can follow.

Treatments for Other Cancers Can Affect the Brain

The drugs (chemotherapies) that are used to treat various forms of cancer can also cause problems with brain function. These anticancer drugs act by poisoning rapidly growing cells; when given for long periods of time they also can poison normally growing cells. Each agent used for chemotherapy works against its own spectrum of cancers. Likewise, each has its own spectrum of side effects, many of which involve the brain and nerves.

The most common problem is a loss of function to the nerves of the legs, leading to numbness in the feet, a burning sensation, pain, and weakness. Sometimes these symptoms become severe enough to dictate switching to some other form of anticancer treatment. After treatment is discontinued the symptoms don't get any worse, and they may improve.

Another treatment, radiation, can trigger neurological symptoms, limiting the amount that can be used to treat cancer. The response of normal brain tissue to radiation often does not appear for weeks or months. So when someone with cancer receives radiation, it can be difficult to tell whether the appearance of neurological symptoms some months later stems from the cancer or from the radiation. Careful imaging studies can usually make the distinction.

REMOTE EFFECTS OF CANCER IN OTHER ORGANS ON THE BRAIN

Sometimes, common cancers in areas far from the brain, like those of the breast or the lung, can produce a rather rare result. Patients develop brain-related problems such as difficulty balancing, walking, or thinking, even though careful study demonstrates that the cancer cells have not spread to the brain. Doctors have known for a long time that cancer can cause such problems, but only recently has the mechanism been clarified.

Most people with cancer develop an immune reaction to it. That is, they make antibodies to help control the cancer. But the antibodies that are directed against the cancer can also damage parts of the person's own brain. As the antibodies "recognize" and kill the cancer cells, they sometimes mistakenly "recognize" some of the nerve cells in the brain and try to kill them, too. The symptoms depend on the part of the brain that is being damaged by the antibodies— memory lapses or motor disturbances, for example. The effect is called "remote" because the cancer has not actually spread to the brain; instead it has disrupted the brain's functioning from back at its outpost by triggering this immune response. The presence of specific antibodies in a person's blood can help diagnose this unusual situation. Sometimes when the underlying cancer is found and treated, the situation gets better.

ATTITUDE AND CANCER: BE REALISTIC

Much popular literature expounds on the importance of keeping a positive attitude when dealing with cancer. We certainly concur that people coping with cancer should do everything they can to keep their spirits up. But the number one best way to battle the disease is to get prompt medical treatment and stick to the regimen. Advice on attitude can do patients a serious disservice if it implies that optimism alone can alter the progression of the disease, particularly if patients respond by halting their treatment in favor of untested, fad programs.

Is there something about specific people that makes them more likely to develop cancer or the treatments more likely to work on them? Genetic factors seem to be the important determinants for some cancers, such as cancer of the breast, bowel, or prostate. Genetic factors undoubtedly increase the risk for other types of cancer, including brain tumors. With other cancers, environmental factors, such as smoking for lung cancer and exposure to the sun for melanoma, are the main culprits. But what about someone's personality, mood, or ability to handle stress? Do they make a difference?

The idea that there could be such a thing as a cancer-prone personality has a long history. The ancients suggested that "melancholic" or pessimistic women were more likely to get breast cancer than "sanguine" or optimistic women. In more modern times, Woody Allen said, "I don't get angry, I grow a tumor instead." Attempts by scientists to test these popular conceptions have been inconclusive at best. There is no persuasive evidence that one personality type is any more likely to develop cancer than another. Nor is there evidence that those under stress "get cancer," ... with one possible exception: depression. Cancer occurs more frequently in those with significant depression. That does not prove that depression causes cancer. It may mean that chronically depressed people's behavior is the culprit—a larger percentage of depressed people smoke than is true of the general population.

How a person with cancer handles the illness is a different, more complicated story. A positive attitude, a determination to fight cancer, does not make much difference. On the other hand, depression, feelings of hopelessness, and social isolation can apparently hasten the progression of cancer and shorten survival. The reason is not entirely clear. Most researchers are focussing on the relationship between depression and the body's immune response to cancer, the theory being that those with depression have a weaker immune response.

At present, it is unclear whether vigorous treatment of depression, with medications and psychotherapy, will improve the outcome in cancer. What does appear to improve the outcome is social support. For both women with breast cancer and men and women with melanomas, participation in support groups improves survival by decreasing social isolation and encouraging better compliance with therapy. Beyond that, participation may help relieve the stress associated with cancer and its treatment.

CHAPTER 17

New Options for Parkinson's Disease

Paul, a surgeon, developed a habit of sitting on his right hand when he wasn't using it, because he wanted to hide the fact that his hand was shaking. This shaking involved not only the fingers but also his wrist. It was most apparent when his hand was resting in his lap. When he reached for something, the shaking would disappear, allowing him to continue to make the fine motor movements required in his surgery. Although the shaking was more of a cosmetic problem than an interference with his functioning, Paul worried that he might have early Parkinson's disease. But he knew that things had changed since his medical school days when Parkinson's disease was not treatable, so he quickly consulted a neurologist.

Guy, too, remembers the days when a diagnosis of Parkinson's signaled an across-the-board disability. His grandmother, who lived with his family when he was a small boy, had the disease, and he vividly remembers the motor problems she had. Talking, moving, getting in and out of a chair, and walking all became difficult for her as the disease progressed. In its later stages, she would sit slumped in a chair with an expressionless face, staring without blinking. At times Guy and his brothers thought she was totally "out of it," but she wasn't. She just could not make the movements required to express her feelings or needs. The effects of the disease made an indelible impression. The contrast between Guy's grandmother's experience and the options available to patients now constitutes one of the major advances in medicine.

In 1817, a British physician, James Parkinson, published a small book entitled *An Essay on the Shaking Palsy.* This title describes two of the classical symptoms that have since been associated with the disease bearing his name: shaking (tremor) and lack of movement (palsy).

Parkinson's disease disrupts normal movement in several ways. It produces problems with starting and carrying out movement such as shuffling cards or buttoning buttons. It interferes with the speed of movements by causing rigidity, a stiffness of limbs, and a resistance of joints to movement. And it results in a loss of the balancing mechanisms involved in walking and turning, making many movements difficult to control. Parkinson's disease usually affects the elderly, with increasing incidence after the age of 60. It afflicts more than 1.5 million people in the United States. About 1 in every 400 people in their 50s has the disease, but it is 10 times more common among people over 85 years of age—with some exceptions. For example, for the actor Michael J. Fox the disease began much earlier.

For people of all ages, Parkinson's disease worsens gradually, but the rate of progression can vary widely from one person to another. This is an important point, because many people will know or have heard of someone who has become disabled rather quickly from Parkinson's disease, which will influence their own concept of the disease. What they don't know about is the large number of people whose condition remains mild and treatable disease for many years.

The early symptoms of the disease are all some people ever experience, particularly if they take medication. More commonly, as people progress, the response to treatment becomes unpredictable. Some go on to the phase of severe symptoms where current therapies are less successful—fortunately, this phase applies to a smaller number of individuals.

EARLY SYMPTOMS OF PARKINSON'S DISEASE

Parkinson's disease can begin quite noticeably or in more subtle ways. For example, tremor (the shaking associated with the disease) is an attention getter, usually bringing the patient into the doctor's office for an early diagnosis.

When the Parkinson's tremor first appears, it may be noticeable only part of the time—when the hand is at rest. A person looks down and sees that his or her hand is shaking. The observation itself may make someone quite self-conscious and anxious, but then the anxiety makes the tremor worse. At this stage, using the arm, as when picking up a pencil, generally seems to make the tremor disappear temporarily. Tremor also disappears during sleep.

In this early stage, a person with Parkinson's disease may have only tremor, without any rigidity or difficulty in starting movements. The tremor may also be quite asymmetrical, affecting only one side and not the other, for example. For some reason the tremor is much more likely to involve the hands and not the legs. It may be a problem at night, when the movements of the hand, before falling asleep, can wake up the person's spouse. With most people for whom the tremor is an early symptom, the diagnosis of Parkinson's disease can be made promptly. If the patient doesn't notice the tremor, his family or friends often do and ask what is wrong.

Other symptoms, however, can be more insidious. Some people with Parkinson's disease never have any tremor; instead they have slowness of movement while walking, turning, or making such hand movements as shuffling cards. These problems come on gradually and may be present for months, even years, before the diagnosis of Parkinson's disease is even considered.

Don was a retired inventor whose hobbies were golf and cards. His problem was that he could no longer shuffle the cards. Somehow he couldn't seem to manipulate his fingers. Eventually, his card-playing buddies had to shuffle and deal for him. When Don came to see us, his slowness of movement and lack of facial expression made the diagnosis of Parkinson's disease almost as he walked through the door of the examining room.

Slowness doesn't quite describe the various ways in which movements may change in early Parkinson's disease. A person may develop difficulty with walking and balance but have no other symptoms of the disease. Common early signs include difficulty turning quickly; a lack of swinging of the arms as one walks; decreases in the small movements of the face so the features look impassive, with a decreased rate of blinking; and difficulty swallowing, sometimes producing a tendency to drool. Another tip-off is a person's handwriting: the letters get smaller and smaller, and the words more crowded together. A neurologist often asks the patient to provide examples of his or her handwriting for the past few years. The progressive smallness of the letters can be very telling.

Because these kinds of movement problems are subtle, the patient, the patient's family, and even many physicians tend to dismiss them. This can delay the diagnosis of Parkinson's disease for many months. In our patients, the average time from the first onset of these

Parkinson symptoms and the establishment of the correct diagnosis is almost two years.

The disease's tendency to impair the small muscles around the eyes and mouth, leaving the face immobile and unexpressive, can be a bigger problem than it seems. Because facial expression is a surprisingly important component of communication, the stony countenances of people with Parkinson's (or stroke) can jeopardize relationships with family and friends.

Sneakiest of all is the third major symptom, stiffness and rigidity of joints, which interferes with fine motor control as in buttoning buttons. Some patients have an especially peculiar symptom—sudden freezing episodes.

Bruce, a 70-year-old writer, came into our office accompanied by his wife. He kept his hand on her arm as he shuffled along in a slow, somewhat uncertain way. As he came through the door of our examining room, he suddenly froze. It was as if his feet were sticking to the ground. His wife encouraged him: "Come on, dear, one, two, one, two ..." The man picked up the cadence count and was able to walk to a chair and sit down. Looking up, he smiled and said, "Doc, I've got gear trouble."

What Has Gone Wrong in Parkinson's Disease?

Parkinson's disease vividly exemplifies how a disease process that affects a small number of nerve cells in the brain can alter functions that depend on the integration of many brain regions. Just as a malfunctioning relay switch in an electrical grid can black out a whole area of a city, so, too, Parkinson's disrupts brain regions beyond the one it affects directly. Parkinson's kills a small group of nerve cells, those in a part of the brain called the substantia nigra. These nerve cells normally produce the neurotransmitter dopamine, which influences the parts of the brain that control movement. As more and more nerve cells in the substantia nigra die, they produce less and less of this chemical; this in turn affects more and more aspects of movement. When one looks at the remaining nerve cells under a microscope, they often contain clumps of material called Lewy Bodies, which look like a bull's-eye. Recent evidence suggests that a protein called alpha synuclein makes up the Lewy Bodies and that genetic abnormalities in this protein are involved in the death of the nerve cells in the substantia nigra.

Genetics and Parkinson's Disease

About a third of people who get Parkinson's disease have a family history of it. However, only a few families show a clear-cut pattern of inheritance. In these rare families, individuals of different generations typically develop the disease at a relatively early age and suffer a more rapid than normal progression, with more severe symptoms. Genetic studies of these families have recently revealed that they carry an abnormal form of a gene that makes alpha synuclein. A second gene, called Parkin, may play a role in individuals who develop Parkinson's disease early in life but have no clear-cut family history. These discoveries have changed scientists' thinking about the mechanism of the disease and may provide the basis for better treatments in the future.

Nongenetic Risk Factors for Parkinson's Disease

For the vast majority of the people with Parkinson's disease, genes are probably not the whole story. In addition to the fact that Parkinson's disease becomes more common as people get older, environmental factors, such as living in a rural community, drinking of well water, and exposure to pesticides may also play roles. However, no specific toxic substance has been identified as contributing to Parkinson's disease. If there are specific risks from the environment, they likely produce the disease in those who are genetically at higher risk to get it.

Treatment of Early Parkinson's Disease

The treatment of Parkinson's disease is one of the great success stories of contemporary medicine. The breakthrough has been based on either replacing or augmenting the missing neurotransmitter, dopamine.

Sinemet is the drug most commonly used for treating Parkinson's disease. It is converted into dopamine in the brain and can be strikingly successful against the disease. Sinemet combines L-DOPA, the substance the brain turns into dopamine, plus an inhibitor that keeps L-DOPA from being broken down in the liver. There is no question that Sinemet alleviates the symptoms of the disease and allows many patients to live useful lives for years. Because Sinemet does have side effects, neurologists usually start with low doses and gradually build up the dose as necessary. The trick is to use the least possible amount of medication and still produce the beneficial effect. A longer acting form of Sinemet, called SinemetCR, allows a patient to take fewer doses of medicine at longer intervals, four to six hours apart instead of three to four hours apart with regular Sinemet. The long-acting form also helps to smooth the effect of the drug, so that a person doesn't experience a sudden peak effect and then a drop-off in effectiveness toward the end of the dosing period.

Sometimes a person's response to Sinemet can help make the diagnosis of Parkinson's disease. For example, if a person is having trouble walking or typing but the cause is not clear we will give Sinemet for three or four weeks. If the symptoms improve, we know it's Parkinson's.

The first phases of treatment with drugs such as Sinemet may last many months or even years. During this time a person will appear normal—even to the trained eye of a physician familiar with Parkinson's disease. But gradually other symptoms may occur, usually a worsening of the original ones. The tremor, which originally involved only one hand, may come to involve both; stiffness while walking may increase; facial mobility may decline; or the person may develop difficulty getting in and out of a chair. Altering the dose of Sinemet—either increasing the dosage or giving medication at more frequent intervals, or perhaps both—can usually moderate these new or increasing symptoms.

SIDE EFFECTS OF SINEMET

Too high a dose of Sinemet can cause confusion and even hallucinations, usually visual and often very striking, in many patients. They see animals or people who appear funny shaped (for instance, very small) or oddly colored (pink or purple). People on Sinemet usually can describe their hallucinations in great detail; they often know these hallucinations are not real, and may not find them particularly disturbing. But this is not always the case. One woman thought she saw little people playing in her driveway. She was very concerned that when her husband drove home from work he would run over them. Other patients can find the hallucinations even more frightening. One patient awoke at night and saw people in his house who were not there, and actually called the police.

More commonly, overdosages of Sinemet cause extra body movements called dyskinesias. The patient just can't keep his or her legs, arms, or lips still, and makes unusual writhing movements while walking. These extra movements can be quite disabling.

In recent years, neurologists have tended not to use Sinemet as the first drug for treatment, but rather a drug that works through the receptor on nerve cells for dopamine. That is a drug, called an agonist, that acts as if it is dopamine. There is a group of these agents including Permax, Requip, and bromocryptine. The major advantage is that they are less likely to induce the extra movements, the dyskinesias. On the other hand, in general they are not as effective in treating the Parkinsonian symptoms. We tend to use one of the agonists in younger patients or milder cases, and Sinemet in older patients, or more severe cases.

When to Treat Early Parkinson's Disease

Even a firm diagnosis of Parkinson's disease doesn't necessarily mean treatment must begin. We commonly ask our patient, "How much is this disease altering your life?" The Parkinson's tremor makes some people so self-conscious that they avoid social situations and become reclusive and often find themselves somewhat depressed. Early treatment can help these people. Others prefer to tolerate the inconvenience of not moving as easily and smoothly as they would like in exchange for Sinemet's side effects.

For the majority of patients the benefits of medications start to wear off after five to eight years, but some patients' symptoms remain responsive to medication for much longer, even to the end of life.

Bruce, the writer with "gear trouble," was one who did very well. He required a rather low dose of Sinemet for 15 years. He still had these peculiar freezing episodes, as, for instance, when he and his wife went to the theater. At intermission, they would get up to go to the lobby. As the crowd of people in the aisle surrounded him, he suddenly would be unable to move. But because Parkinson's causes problems in initiating movement and is not a form of paralysis, all his wife had to do was touch him gently on the arm and quietly say, "One, two, one, two." This mild stimulus was enough to break the "freeze" and get him moving again. So while he still had his "gear trouble," the rest of him did fine on rather low doses of Sinemet.

Day-to-Day Changes in the Symptoms of Parkinson's Disease

Almost everyone with Parkinson's disease has good days and bad days. Stress, fatigue, and an illness such as the flu can easily send a Parkinson's patient on a downswing. We all live our lives with a certain amount of stress, but those with Parkinson's disease have a special "stress barometer." When symptoms get acutely worse for no apparent reason, they should take a look at how they are living. Instead of trying to adjust medications during these times, it is better to ride things out and try to modify, or at least recognize, these complicating factors.

Psychological Issues and Early Parkinson's Disease

Many people with Parkinson's resist accepting that they have a new, lifelong condition that calls for psychological adjustments and changes in lifestyle. So we spend a lot of time talking with patients about several types of concerns.

Preconceived Notions about Parkinson's Disease

Parkinson's disease is common, and many of us already are strongly influenced by reports of people who have become invalids. This is particularly true of older people whose previous experience with the disease might have been at a time when there was no treatment. The treatments available today have extended life expectancy by 10 to 15 years, many of which are very good years. In addition, every year there are new medications and approaches. What was once a dismal picture is now one of hope and advancement.

Problems with Being Dependent on Medicine

Having to depend on medicine is both a literal and psychological problem. It can seem as if one's life revolves around taking a little pill, and many people find that very tough. This is one of the most common problems we encounter when first treating a person who has just received the diagnosis of Parkinson's disease. That little pill is a two-edged sword. On one hand, it is essential for optimal functioning. On the other hand, a person is giving up his independence since every few hours he must take his medication or symptoms will come back. We see this in almost all people who need to take medicines on a regular basis, not just those with Parkinson's disease. Early on, in fact, it is not unusual for people to keep experimenting to see whether they really need their medication; sometimes they even stop taking it. They may not notice a difference for two or three days, but then the symptoms will return, often worse than they seemed before. If a dose is missed, it's important to remember not to try to make it up. There is a time lag before the effect of Sinemet is noticeable, and it is easier to overdose oneself than to see any effect of temporary under-dosage. Fortunately, most people learn after doing this once or twice that they really must take the medication.

Another problem is the chance of forgetting to take the medication on schedule or difficulty remembering having taken it. A lot of tricks can help keep things straight. The easiest is to have a pill box containing each day's medication and to keep it near the toothbrush as a reminder at the end of the day to put in the next day's supply. Drug companies also sometimes provide boxes for an entire week's supply of medication, with each day and time of day labeled.

Uncertainty about the Future in Parkinson's Disease

A vague and uncertain future scares many patients. What will happen to me? Will I become an invalid? We think physicians should be candid. We always tell a person what to expect, and what may happen. Each person is, of course, different, and there may be different answers at different stages of the disease. But on the whole, Parkinson's disease does not suddenly change its clinical course for any given individual. It is reasonably predictable. The person who has had a slowly progressive process, for example, only involving tremor of one hand, will probably do very well—going many years of being responsive to medicines. On the other hand, a few unfortunate people experience the onset of the disease at a relatively young age and suffer a rapidly progressive course. In other words, a given person's pattern is predictable. What is not predictable is one person's course versus another's.

THE INTERMEDIATE PHASE OF PARKINSON'S DISEASE

Physicians call the second phase of Parkinson's the "brittle" phase. This refers to the fact that the patient's response to medications can be unstable during this period. The term "brittle" was first used to describe people with diabetes who required very close monitoring of their dosage of insulin. With the medications for Parkinson's disease, the range between underdosage and overdosage can be narrow. Patients often have wide swings between the two extremes, sometimes very rapidly.

Clarence came into the examining room making very abnormal movements as he walked. His head was twisting to one side, his arms flung around in a disjointed way, and he lurched from side to side. We wanted to reach out and grab him before he hurt himself. He sat down, smiled, and said, "I'm a little hyper today." Over the next 40 minutes, all these movements abated and he was able to sit quietly. Forty minutes later, he was very stiff and couldn't get out of his chair. When he leaned forward, he would have fallen over if we had not caught him.

When he was underdosed, Clarence was rigid and slow moving, and his tremor became prominent. When he was overdosed, he had extra movements, twisting of the limbs or mouth, constant chewing movements, and an inability to keep his legs still. Clarence could easily recognize when he was underdosed and did not like it. He could not move. He also couldn't think quite correctly. He called it being in a "brain fog." In contrast, in the overdosed state he didn't recognize how much he was moving. All he knew was that he could move quite easily. Like many people with Parkinson's disease, Clarence would rather be overdosed than underdosed. But by carefully monitoring his medication, we found the balance point.

Treatment of the Intermediate Phase of Parkinson's Disease

Treating Parkinson's disease in its intermediate phase is an art, with a little science thrown in. The first line of defense is to adjust the existing medications. Primarily this means larger doses at closer intervals. But no two patients are the same. Nor is this year's adjustment for a person necessarily going to be correct next year. It is a constant process of trial and error, with two rules as a guide. First, don't change things too fast. It takes time for a change of medication to have an effect. It is important for an individual to know this, and not to become impatient.

Second, don't change two things at once. Medications have interactions. If problems surface after a simultaneous change in two different medications, it's it is hard to figure out which one is responsible. For example, we try not to change the dose of Sinemet and add an antidepressant medication at the same time. If things do not go well, we won't know whether one medicine or the combination of both is at fault. It is much easier to determine how to proceed in the future if it is clear which change in medication is the critical one.

Don, the retired inventor, did quite well with his Parkinson's medication for about eight years, then he began "running out of gas."

About three hours after a dose of Sinemet, his symptoms would come back, and he would be very stiff, almost unable to walk. Several different changes in the timing and combination of medications eventually made clear that he had to take medicine every three hours while awake to keep functioning. This was some years ago. Now we would prescribe one of the new add-on medications, such as Permax, that can smooth out the effects of Sinemet in some people.

Diet and Parkinson's Disease

Once upon a time, physicians tried to adjust a person's diet while taking Sinemet. The idea was that proteins from an ordinary diet would interfere with the absorption of the medication and the passage of L-DOPA into the brain. In one extreme diet, patients ate only one protein-containing meal a day, at night. Time has shown that this approach does not work for most people. Rather, it is important to take medications in as consistent a relationship to meals as possible, and not take medication before lunch one day and after lunch the next. But the patient can eat every kind of food, and neither alcohol nor vitamins appear to affect the disease one way or another. Some evidence suggests that vitamin E may protect against the occurrence of Parkinson's disease, but no evidence shows that it has any effect once the disease is present.

One of the exciting lines of research in Parkinson's disease is the role of abnormalities in metabolism, specifically, in the function of small packets of enzymes called mitochondria. Mitochondria are found in all cells that are involved in the metabolism of sugar to produce energy. In Parkinson's disease, mitochondria in specific cells of the brain may be abnormal. A protective factor for these mitochondria is a substance called co-enzyme Q10 (sometimes called vitamin Q10). Studies are trying to determine if co-enzyme Q10 can have a beneficial effect in this disease.

THE LATE PHASE OF PARKINSON'S DISEASE

In the late stage of Parkinson's the medications are no longer as effective for some patients, and the lack of movement may become disabling. A person may have difficulty rolling over in bed, getting out of a chair, or starting to walk. Like the patient with "gear trouble," he or she may freeze, suddenly becoming unable to move. The fluctuations in response to medicine occur at more frequent intervals. The normal movements used to maintain balance, called postural reflexes, may be lost. As patients start to lose their balance, they may not be able to catch themselves and may fall. Falling is a particular hazard when getting out of a chair or getting up from bed.

One of our patients developed a particular problem walking her dog. The dog would see another dog and start to take off, pulling her off balance. After a few falls, which fortunately did not result in any injuries, she turned these dog-walking duties over to her husband.

Some people have a very distinctive symptom. They start walking, quite slowly, taking very small steps, but as they lean forward, they throw themselves off balance and begin walking faster and faster, unable to stop. If not caught by someone else, they can crash into the wall or furniture.

Treating the Late Phase of Parkinson's Disease

Current medical treatments are not very effective for people in the late phase of Parkinson's disease. The basic problem is that the disease progressively kills more and more nerve cells in the substantia nigra. Eventually not enough nerve cells remain to respond to the L-DOPA. This calls for completely different strategies, such as surgery, perhaps even including transplantation of brain tissue.

Seeking Better Treatments for the Late Phase of Parkinson's Disease

In trying to understand a disease process in human beings, simulating the disease in another animal can be crucial. An animal model, as scientists call it, provides a way of testing new therapies and techniques without endangering human patients. Usually, finding such a model takes endless hours in the laboratory. However, sometimes a model falls into one's lap. But the scientist has to have the imagination to see it sitting there.

An unusual chain of events led to the best animal model for Parkinson's disease. It started when a young man in his 20s came to a physician's office with classical symptoms of Parkinson's disease. Knowing that Parkinson's disease is primarily a disease of the elderly, the physician was curious enough to question the young man in detail about any medications or drugs he had taken. The patient confessed to having taken an experimental street drug a few weeks before called MPTP, which was an illicit copy of the painkiller Demerol.

It didn't take long to figure out that MPTP was a poison that could trigger Parkinson's disease. When taken by mouth, it is selectively toxic to exactly the same cells in the substantia nigra that are affected in classical Parkinson's disease. This amazing series of observations transformed research in Parkinson's disease for a variety of reasons. First, the fact that a toxin, or poison (MPTP), can produce the disease raised the question of whether toxins in our environment that are similar to MPTP might be the cause of the classical forms of Parkinson's disease in the general population. So far, extensive studies of the histories of patients with Parkinson's disease have not revealed any common pattern of exposure to drugs or chemicals, with the possible exception of pesticides.

But the observations by the physician did provide the long-sought animal model for this disease. Animals given MPTP developed Parkinson's disease. The whole approach to the surgical treatments we now use is based on being able to produce Parkinson's disease in a monkey and then making the disease better with precise surgery or transplanted cells.

Surgical Strategies for Parkinson's Disease

The biggest change in treating late-stage Parkinson's disease is the return of surgical procedures. Two groups of people are the best candidates for this surgery: those with a severe tremor that does not respond to medicines; and those who are having the extra movements, the "dyskinesias" associated with over-response to medication.

Surgical procedures to modify Parkinson's disease were originally tried over 50 years ago, but such early surgical approaches were abandoned for two reasons. First, the success of L-DOPA, a medical therapy, made surgery unnecessary for many patients. Second, the surgical techniques, which required making small deliberate areas of injury in the brain (known as a surgical lesion) were too inaccurate, and often resulted in unintended damage. The development of two technologies changed that. Brain imaging can now determine exactly where to put the surgical probe in order to make the lesion. And surgeons can now use a probe to record the very distinctive patterns of signals sent from particular brain cells, thus guiding them to the correct spot.

Neurosurgeons are currently using three surgical approaches: Stereotactic surgery, which is the process of making very tiny lesions in just the right place in the brain; electrical stimulation of the brain, in which a "pacemaker" is placed in areas to control motor movements, much as a cardiac pacemaker stabilizes heartbeat; and transplantation of tissue into the brain.

STEREOTACTIC SURGERY

The control of motor movements is a balance between positive and negative signals from the brain. When you reach for a cup of coffee, for example, some muscles are commanded to move, and others are commanded not to move. Parkinson's disease puts these control mechanisms out of whack. The goal of surgery is to neutralize the part of the brain that is causing excess movements. To do this, a probe, no bigger than a pencil lead, is carefully introduced into the brain, under the guidance of three-dimensional images provided by imaging techniques, such as CT or MRI scans. In addition, many neurosurgeons use a probe from which they can also record. When they get to their target—a specific group of nerve cells deep within the brain—the electrical signals recorded from that probe change, telling the surgeons the probe is exactly where they want it to be—sometimes in a part of the brain called the thalamus, and at other times in an area called the globus pallidus. Thus, this surgery is sometimes called a thalamotomy or a pallidotomy.

The results of this stereotactic surgical approach can be spectacular, particularly for the relief of tremor. A patient who can barely control his hand may have an immediate beneficial result, and walk out of the hospital a few days later able to write or bring a cup of coffee up to his lips.

The tremor of Paul, the surgeon, particularly the tremor of his right hand, responded to Sinemet for about two years. Then his response to the medication began to fluctuate unpredictably. Sometimes he would have tremor; at others times he would have medication-induced twitches not only of his hands but also his legs, face, and mouth. Paul had to stop performing surgery and was able to lead a semblance of a normal life for only a few hours each day. Paul and his doctor decided it was time to try stereotactic surgery.

An MRI of Paul's brain permitted the neurosurgeon to identify the landmarks (the coordinates) that he would use to guide the probe to the exact location at which to make the lesion. Paul was then taken to the operating room. While he was still awake and under local anesthesia, surgeons drilled a small hole in his skull. (It is possible to do this type of surgery, because the brain has no pain sensation.) Very slowly, the surgeon moved a probe into the left side of Paul's brain. Recordings from the probe emitted a constant series of beeps that sound like static. Different parts of the brain emit different sequences of beeps, serving as audible signposts. Finally, the beeps indicted that the neurosurgeon was at the spot identified by the imaging studies. By putting an electric current through the probe, the surgeon made a small lesion, no larger than the end of an eraser on a pencil. The excessive heat destroyed the cells causing the symptoms. The tremor of Paul's right hand immediately decreased. Paul could hardly believe what had happened. His hand had not been that steady for years. He went home five days after his surgery.

Over the next few months, Paul had much less trouble with his medications. He no longer suffered the wide swings of responses to the drugs and actually decreased the amount he was taking by about one half. One year later, he still showed the beneficial effects of the procedure. He did not go back to performing surgery himself, but still plays a valuable role in teaching. At times he stands right behind a young surgeon and essentially guides him or her through an operation.

QUESTIONS ABOUT SURGERY FOR PARKINSON'S DISEASE

How successful is this surgery? For those with a tremor from Parkinson's disease, it is successful about 85 percent of the time, and for those with essential tremor, about 50 percent of the time. Drug-induced movements, the dyskinesias, also may respond quite well. On the other hand, slowness of movement and problems with walking and balance are much less likely to be influenced by surgery.

The major limitation of this surgical approach has to do with its potential effects on being able to speak. If a lesion is made on both sides of the brain, a person's understanding of what others are saying and the ability to know what he or she wants to say will both be fine, as will be the ability to write or use a computer. The only impairment is inability to speak. Consequently, surgery is performed on only one side, returning functioning to the other side of the body. If a person is having a tremor of both hands, the surgery is usually done on the left side so that the use of the dominant hand, usually the right hand, will be returned to function. (Because things are crossed in the brain, the control of motor movement for a right-handed person is usually on the left side.)

Refinements to this surgery are extending the benefits to include more of the Parkinson's symptoms. In the late 1990s another small group of nerve cells, the subthalamic nucleus, became the target for the surgical lesion. Careful studies of stereotactic surgery in animals with Parkinson's disease indicated that a lesion in this small area was even more effective than the usual lesion in the globus pallidus or thalamus. The surgeon's ability to hit such a small target results directly from the advances in imaging techniques; such pinpoint accuracy would have been impossible just a few years ago. Results of this new surgery are very encouraging because more of the symptoms of Parkinson's disease respond to this therapy.

BRAIN STIMULATION FOR PARKINSON'S DISEASE

Another advance in surgery has a science-fiction sounding name: deep brain stimulation. In this technique, first developed in Europe and now increasingly used in the United States, the surgeon does not make a surgical lesion. Instead, a small electrode is implanted into the brain in one of the same places where stereotactic lesions would be made (the globus pallidus or the subthalamic nucleus). The electrode emits an electrical current, interrupting the abnormal signals that cause the Parkinsonian symptoms, particularly tremor. Unlike a lesion, which destroys the target group of brain cells, the stimulator disrupts signals in a reversible way. It remains in the brain; its electrical pulse can be adjusted in the doctor's office as needed, even turned off at times. The stimulator can be placed on both sides of the brain, relieving symptoms on both sides of the body without affecting the ability to speak. As with stereotactic surgery, the immediate results can be spectacular.

An implanted stimulator has one potential problem: the risk of infection. The brain does not like to have foreign things like wires left in it. Fortunately, infections happen rarely (in fewer than three patients out of a hundred) and can usually be treated with antibiotics and cured. Comparison studies between making a surgical lesion and implanting a stimulator indicate a greater decrease in symptoms with a stimulator, with fewer complications. In just a few years, deep brain stimulation has become the preferred treatment for Parkinson's disease, primarily for those whose tremor and dyskinesias do not respond to medications.

Brain Tissue Transplantation for Parkinson's Disease

The newest therapeutic approach is the transplantation into the brain of tissue that can provide the needed transmitter, dopamine. The goal of this surgical procedure is for the transplanted tissue to ultimately make connections to existing nerve cells and provide dopamine to the brain in much the same way that a medicine would, only in a more longlasting manner. Originally, surgeons removed part of the patient's own adrenal gland, which could be a source for dopamine, and placed it in the brain. However, the adrenal tissue did not survive very well. The next approach was to obtain the substantia nigra from the brain of a human fetus. As with the adrenal gland, this tissue was placed in the brain of the patients. The results with the fetal tissue are still being evaluated. Thus far the period of follow-up has been short, less than a few years for most patients. However a few individuals have had fetal transplants that have functioned for at least 10 years. It is not clear whether this form of therapy will have a place in the treatment of Parkinson's disease.

For some of these patients the transplants have been too successful. For about a year new cells seem to be helping, but then symptoms in keeping with too much dopamine begin to appear. Patients have increasing problems with dyskinesias that can be quite disabling. Many unknowns surround the approach of transplanting cells into the brain. How much tissue is enough? What can help the tissue to survive? What measures can control its actions?

The latest controversy is over the use of human embryonic stem cells. These cells are removed from a very early embryo produced by fertilization in a dish in a laboratory, in vitro fertilization, or IVF. These early cells have the potential to develop into any tissue in the body—including nerve cells of the brain.

Some scientists believe that stem cells will be a source for nerve cells to "cure" Parkinson's disease. We don't think it will be that easy. The same questions about the amount, survival, and control of transplanted tissue also apply to stem cells. Other problems include how to get the stem cells to become nerve cells and provide the correct neurotransmitter (dopamine), and how to prevent them from forming other types of cells, even tumors. It's an exciting area of research, but much remains to be done. This approach may someday be used to treat Parkinson's disease, but that day is five to ten years down the line.

PREVENTIVE STRATEGIES FOR PARKINSON'S DISEASE

The current approach to therapy, the replacement of the missing neurotransmitter, treats the symptoms but does not alter the underlying disease process. The real progress will come when researchers also learn how to prevent the progression of the disease. The goal is to prevent the degeneration of the nerve cells at the site of attack, the substantia nigra. Several approaches to altering the actual progression of the disease are under scrutiny. Two agents, vitamin E and Deprenyl (or Eldepryl), can reportedly slow the progression of Parkinson's disease. These claims are based on evidence from experimental animals exposed to MPTP. Even though some evidence suggests that those taking vitamin E are less likely to get Parkinson's disease, vitamin E did not appear to have any effect on the disease's progression once it began.

Deprenyl is more controversial. Research in animals originally raised hopes that it would be the first agent to actually slow down the progression of the disease, but the initial enthusiasm for Deprenyl seems to be waning. It may delay the onset of symptoms that are difficult to treat with current medications, such as problems with balance and falling. But it is not the magic bullet that doctors and patients would like, although it may be a first step.

In the laboratory, there is some indication that dopamine agonists, such as Permax or Requip, may have neuroprotective effects in animal models of Parkinson's disease. The jury is still out as to whether this is true for the human disease. However, this possible neuroprotective effect is one of the reasons that some neurologists initiate therapy with one of these agonists, either alone or in combination with Sinemet.

Another area of research is the potential use of substances called trophic factors, which promote the development and survival of certain groups of nerve cells in the brain. Trophic factors can also help damaged nerve cells recover. Different populations of nerve cells use specific trophic factors that go by acronyms, like NGF or BDNF, relating to their biological action. The aim is to find the specific trophic factors that will protect the nerve cells in the substantia nigra that are attacked by Parkinson's disease. A number of pharmaceutical companies are testing these substances in experimental animals. It is too early to tell if these trophic factors will provide an effective new approach to treatment.

NONMOTOR MANIFESTATIONS OF PARKINSON'S DISEASE

Most people think of Parkinson's as an illness involving problems of motor control, but there can be other problems, too. A very bright scientist we know had the motor symptoms of his Parkinson's disease under reasonable control, but his thinking and speech were very slow and halting. When answering a question he would stop in mid-sentence for what seemed like minutes (in actuality 30 to 40 seconds), and then continue. Many of his colleagues thought he was becoming demented. Not so; rather, his speed of processing information, like his motor movements, was slow and sometimes "froze." Fortunately, with some adjustments of his medication, he improved markedly.

Dementia and Parkinson's Disease

About one-fifth of those with this disease can have true dementia; that is, progressive problems with thinking, remembering, and speaking. Some of these people appear to have two disorders: a combination of Parkinson's disease and Alzheimer's disease, with Alzheimer's disease causing the problems with memory and other mental abilities. However, some people with Parkinson's disease and dementia may not show the brain changes characteristic of Alzheimer's disease.

These patients differ from classical Parkinson patients in that they are much less likely to respond well to the usual medications. They are also unusually sensitive to these medications and more likely to have hallucinations and other behavioral abnormalities. When the brains of these people are examined under a microscope, however, the nerve cells throughout the brain contain the same Lewy Bodies (those clumps of abnormal material that look like bull's-eyes) as do people with Parkinson's disease. Thus, the patients are said to have "Lewy Body dementia." It is not clear if this is just a variant of Parkinson's disease or a different disease with Parkinsonian features.

Communication and Parkinson's Disease

In the early phase of Parkinson's disease, a person may have difficulty projecting his voice. One man, for example, had difficulty getting up and speaking at a meeting of salespeople. He couldn't seem to speak loud enough. He solved the problem by always using a portable microphone. Patients for whom tremor is a prominent part of the disease may experience a tremor of the voice as well.

As the disease progresses, slowness of movement can effect how the tongue, lips, and palate move. A person can become increasingly hard to understand. Later in the disease, the brain's ability to process language may slow down, and patients cannot think of what they want to say as quickly as they could before. In the late stages of Parkinson's disease, Guy's grandmother was almost mute. Her understanding of what was said to her was fine; it was the output that was at fault. People caring for a person with advanced Parkinson's disease often make the error of assuming that because a person does not speak, that person does not understand. People may say things in front of an individual that they would never say under normal circumstances, to everyone's detriment. It is best to assume that the person with advanced Parkinson's disease hears and understands everything you say.

Depression and Parkinson's Disease

As many as one-half of all patients with Parkinson's disease also have depression. This may seem an obvious response to their illness. Their lives have changed, they are not sure what will happen, they are now dependent on taking medicines at regular intervals, and they often have had contact with other patients who have more severe symptoms, so they are worried about their futures. All of this is frightening and upsetting. However, depression may be more than a purely psychological reaction. It's possible that the chemical changes that occur in the disease itself specifically lead to depression.

Physicians often miss the presence of depression in Parkinson's disease. They miss the fact that people have trouble controlling their emotions, that they become teary much more easily. That is unfortunate, because proper treatment of the accompanying depression can have strikingly positive results, making the treatment of Parkinson's disease much easier. Drugs such as Paxil or Zoloft, or sometimes Prozac, are often used for the treatment of the mood disorder, and do not interfere with the anti-Parkinson drugs.

Hallucinations and Parkinson's Disease

As the disease progresses, some people have hallucinations, usually visual, that are much more intense and disturbing than those we discussed earlier. This kind of problem is one of the more common reasons many people with Parkinson's disease may require nursing homes for their care.

From a motor standpoint, Walt's Parkinson's disease was not all that bad. He had some tremor and stiffness, but required rather low doses of Sinemet. In the fourth year of his disease he suddenly began having vivid hallucinations of people in his house. One night he awoke to see a person in the chair in his room. He even carried the rather heavy chair downstairs, near the front door. When the person would not leave, Walt called the police. The police were able to assure him that there was nobody there. We treated him with low doses of Clozapine, and the hallucinations got much better. They were not entirely gone, but they were not nearly as frightening.

Clozapine is commonly used for treating schizophrenia. People with Parkinson's disease can be exquisitely sensitive to this drug, requiring only about one-tenth the dose used in those with schizophrenia.

Blood Pressure and Parkinson's Disease

People with Parkinson's usually have lower blood pressure than others. And the anti-Parkinson medications tend to lower blood pressure even more. Thus, some patients may have trouble with low blood pressure, particularly when they first try to stand—a phenomenon known as orthostatic hypotension. When they stand, their blood pressure drops, and not enough blood is pumped to the brain. They feel light-headed and dizzy and think they are about to faint. In extreme cases, they may actually faint.

The answer, simply, is to be very careful about standing up suddenly. When getting out of bed, it is best to sit on the edge first for a few minutes and wiggle the feet before standing. For more severe problems, adding salt to the diet, taking Florinef (a drug that helps retain salt), or using elastic stockings to keep blood from pooling in the legs, can help boost blood pressure. Some people will respond to even one of these measures, others require all three.

Sexual Function and Parkinson's Disease

Because physicians and patients alike can be embarrassed to broach the subject, sexual problems in Parkinson's are often ignored. The sudden appearance of the drug Viagra has changed all that, at least for men.

Many men with Parkinson's disease are impotent; that is, they have difficulty achieving and maintaining an erection. Whether this results from the underlying disease or the side effects of medication is not clear. Impotence may also result from depression or the use of medications for depression. It is too early to tell if Viagra will be an effective drug for men or women with Parkinson's disease, but many of our patients are trying it. Viagra is still a new drug, and much remains unknown about its vagaries and side effects. So close monitoring by a physician is advised. For more on Viagra, see Chapter 8, "Bodily Functions and Your Brain."

PARKINSON'S DISEASE PLUS

Several diseases share some of the symptoms of Parkinson's disease plus other symptoms, such as difficulty moving one's eyes, or low blood pressure. Though these related conditions are much rarer, the broader term "Parkinson Syndrome" is sometimes used to cover all bases. These other diseases are less likely to respond to anti-Parkinson medications like Sinemet, perhaps because the disease process is more widespread, extending in the brain beyond the substantia nigra.

FUTURE TREATMENTS AND PREVENTION OF PARKINSON'S DISEASE

A new experimental approach to transplantation takes advantage of the techniques of modern genetic engineering. The idea is that cells from a person's brain would be given the genetic machinery to make dopamine, and then placed back in the brain. Researchers have developed this procedure in monkeys with Parkinson's disease, and may begin studying it in people. If successful, this procedure would avoid the controversial question of using human fetal tissue to treat the disease.

Just in the last year there has been increasing interest in the possible use of stem cells, and the possibility that they can form dopamine-producing nerve cells. Scientists are just at the beginning stages of research with these cells to determine if they will be suitable for transplantation, first in the animal models of Parkinson's disease and then in human volunteers.

Treating Parkinson's disease by replacing a missing neurotransmitter or transplanting nerve cells does not get at the basic question about the disease—why a specific set of nerve cells dies. The answer to this question may come from new genetic information. Using modern genetic techniques, researchers have transplanted the abnormal gene for making alpha synuclein into a variety of experimental animals, including fruit flies and mice. This increased the production of this protein in the animals, which killed the nerve cells that use dopamine as the animals got older. These dying nerve cells had accumulations of alpha synuclein very similar to that found in Lewy Bodies in people with Parkinson's disease. These experiments have shifted the focus from replacing dying nerve cells to altering the accumulation of alpha synuclein.

The ultimate goal is to prevent Parkinson's disease by identifying and treating people before the symptoms become full blown. In order to do this, scientists need to know who is at risk. At present, no one knows know how to identify these people, but some leads have surfaced. For example, researchers are following those exposed to the few identified environmental risks for Parkinson's disease, such as pesticides. Thus, for example, researchers can follow migrant agricultural workers to see if they begin to develop the symptoms of Parkinson's disease, so they can be treated early.

The scientific approach to Parkinson's disease follows the same path as for Alzheimer's disease. Leads from genetics may result in ideas about the basic mechanism of the disease, lighting the way for new approaches to treatment. The loss of specific groups of nerve cells starts long before—probably years before—any symptoms appear. The challenge is to detect the diseases in their early stages and block their advance.

WHAT YOU CAN DO TO COPE WITH PARKINSON'S DISEASE: THE IMPORTANCE OF ATTITUDE AND LIFESTYLE

Medications and surgery for Parkinson's disease represent one of the major advances in medicine, but keep in mind that some of your best defenses against the disease are in your own hands.

- *Seek out support.* Being diagnosed with a chronic illness can be overwhelming, and it's understandable that feelings of anger, or "why me?" will follow. Though these feelings are counterproductive if they go on too long, acknowledging and discussing them is a vital step in dealing with illness. Patients may not be able to handle these feelings all by themselves; discussions with a counselor or with groups of other patients may be of enormous help. The worst thing a person can do is to go into a shell, withdrawing from usual activities and social contacts. A cycle of anxiety over what people will think, more stress and more symptoms, and often an accompanying depression, make things worse. It is important, for example, to keep working as long as possible. We have been impressed over the years with the fact that those who don't let the disease get them down, who don't withdraw from their familiar activities, do much better. They seem to be more responsive to their medications and less likely to be depressed.

- *Don't try to hide the disease.* We have seen many people try to hide the fact that they have Parkinson's disease, swearing their families to secrecy. That doesn't work. The disease is too obvious, and trying to hide it only leads to more embarrassment and stress between the person with the disease and his or her colleagues and friends.

- *Exercise.* The stiffness and rigidity of Parkinson's disease leads some people to become very sedentary. Others have a fear of falling that limits their activities. Numerous studies show that exercise programs not only improve movements and balance but also make those with Parkinson's disease feel much better about themselves. One of the most important things you can do is to develop an exercise program that maintains your joint mobility, balance, and posture. Start with exercises that will put your major joints (ankles, knees, hips, spine, shoulders, elbows, and wrists) through a full range of motion. Nothing fancy, just make these body parts move. Walking on a regular schedule is an excellent idea. Some find that when they first start to walk, they are slow and hesitant. However, after they get warmed up, they do very well. Swimming is also an excellent exercise because it requires very little balance and gravity is not a factor. Most of the exercises we recommend are the same type most people would do simply to maintain good mobility. In addition, a few have been designed specifically for Parkinson's disease.

The Appendix provides information about exercises that aid the specific problems related to walking, getting out of a chair, facial movements, and other symptoms.

- *Stay informed.* Many pharmaceutical companies are trying to develop newer treatments for Parkinson's disease. The media regularly trumpet potential breakthroughs. Add the vast amount of information available on the Internet and it becomes difficult to separate the wheat from the chaff. It is important to develop reliable sources of information, either a physician or a support group that provides accurate information or answers to questions. Several national foundations concerned with Parkinson's disease, as well as many local support groups, can provide solid information.

CHAPTER 18

SHAKING, WEAKNESS, ALS, AND YOUR BRAIN

TREMOR

Even though he was in his eighties, Henry still served as a consultant to the U.S. Navy. During WWII he had worked with the British on the development of radar and was considered a world's expert in this area. Every so often, when the navy had a problem with the radar equipment on one of their large vessels that they could not fix, they called Henry for help. Henry went to the naval vessel, took the equipment apart, and fixed it. There was only one limitation. Henry had a severe tremor any time he tried to do anything with his hands. He could not pick up a cup of coffee, he could not write his name. And, most important in relation to activities for the navy, he could not use a screwdriver. When he was not using his hands, they remained quite still. However, the moment he picked up an object, they started to shake. The harder he tried to quiet them, the harder they shook. On a ship, Henry stood behind a young engineer and talked him through what he wanted done.

Henry had noted that if he had a drink containing alcohol, his hands were much steadier. However, smelling of alcohol while working on a naval vessel was not always acceptable.

Henry had the most common disorder of movement, known as tremor. Tremor refers to a repetitive shaking of the fingers, hands, legs, or even the head, lips, or mouth. Some tremors are very fast, with very fine movements. Under certain circumstances, most of us experience tremor, usually of our hands. This may occur when we are nervous, under stress, drink too much coffee, or are recovering from drinking too much alcohol. It is also common when people are involved in vigorous physical activity. Tremor under these circumstances is normal. Tremors such as Henry's involve much larger, slower movements and usually appear when an individual tries to use his hands. These tremors are not normal.

To control movement, the brain employs a very carefully balanced system on many levels. The brain must coordinate not only the signal to make a movement but also feedback from the moving limb required to regulate the speed, direction, and amount of the movement. When a tremor such as Henry's occurs, these regulating systems go out of sync. This can involve different parts of the brain, but particularly the cerebellum and its connections at the base of the brain.

There are a number of names for the condition Henry had. One name is "benign essential tremor." The name indicates that the tremor does not result from a more serious life-threatening disease, though it can cause considerable difficulty. Another name is "familial tremor," meaning that it runs in families. Finally, the term "senile tremor" emphasizes that it occurs and gets worse late in life. These are all variants of the same condition: a tremor that gradually worsens over the years, and becomes apparent when a person is making a purposeful movement. A good catch-all term that most medical people use is "essential tremor."

Like Henry, people with essential tremor can be sitting quite comfortably and quietly with no tremor, but as soon as they reach to pick something up—like a cup of coffee—their hand starts to shake so much that the contents spill. As the tremor progresses over time, writing a note may become virtually impossible. More rarely, this tremor can involve other parts of the body. Shaking of the head or legs can develop. The movie star Katharine Hepburn developed this kind of tremor many years ago, and her recent films show the progression of this disorder from difficulty with her head to involvement of her voice.

Doctors and laymen alike sometimes mistake this type of tremor for a symptom of Parkinson's disease. Unfortunately, this wastes time and energy, because anti-Parkinson's medications do not work for essential tremor.

Treatment of Essential Tremor

Many people with essential tremor, like Henry, experience a strange phenomenon: they find that their hands settle down with a little alcohol. It doesn't take very much; just half a glass of wine usually does the trick. So when they go out for lunch or dinner, they take a little drink before they go. Then, when they are eating, they happily find that the tremor is damped down. They can cut meat or drink coffee without much difficulty. This is one of the few examples where a little alcohol clearly has a specific, positive effect on how the brain functions.

Medications can also lessen the shaking. One of them is Propranolol, a drug that blocks receptors that send unwanted signals to the brain. Just a small amount each day can keep the tremor under control. However, these medications, even when helpful, may not permit fine motor coordination. Henry, for example, could sign his name when he was taking Propranolol, but still could not use a screwdriver, as he could after drinking alcohol. Both alcohol and Propranolol influence the balancing mechanisms in the cerebellum and its connections.

For those with severe tremor, deep brain stimulation, as is used in Parkinson's disease, may be helpful. The target for stimulation, however, is different in tremor than it is in Parkinson's disease. For tremor, the stimulator is placed in a part of the brain, the thalamus, which moderates how incoming sensory information is processed.

Future Treatments for Essential Tremor

Essential tremor often runs in families, which strongly suggests that an underlying genetic abnormality causes this disorder. However, so far researchers have not identified any candidate genes to support this idea, as they have for Parkinson's disease. Finding a genetic abnormality remains an important goal for the future, because if one can be found, it may lead to understanding the basic mechanism of the disorder.

The two treatments that medicine now uses both emerged from chance observation and not from any basic understanding of the disease. Hopefully, new treatments will be developed as scientists learn more about the underlying cause of the problem. As with other movement disorders, the hope is not only to treat the symptoms, but to prevent the disease process.

ATAXIA

Jay was a hard-driving businessman who retired somewhat involuntarily at the age of 64, when his company was taken over by another. Initially, he frequented his favorite golf courses and seemed to be adjusting to his new life. But gradually, his golf partners noted that his coordination was off. He had difficulty walking along narrow paths between greens and seemed unsteady climbing out of a sand trap. In the locker room, he had to hold the wall when he went to the shower. These symptoms worsened to the point that his friends talked to his wife about their concerns and he sought treatment.

When he was seen by a neurologist, his thinking, memory, and strength all appeared normal, but his coordination was terrible. He could not stand with his feet together. He walked with his legs wide apart and couldn't turn quickly. When he tried to touch the physician's finger with his own he couldn't hit the target. All these symptoms pointed to a condition called ataxia, a term neurologists use to describe a general breakdown of motor control. The next challenge was to find the cause. Long discussions with Jay and his wife eventually revealed that both, but particularly Jay, had been "secret drinkers" for a long time. After his retirement the problem got worse, so that not only did he drink a lot, he ate very little, deriving most of his calories from alcohol. It took some time for Jay to realize that he had a drinking problem, but when he did, he stopped. His ataxia gradually improved, and so did his mental outlook. He joined the board of the local hospital and started teaching a night course on economics at a community college. His gait improved, as did his golf scores. Jay was lucky. His ataxia had an identifiable, treatable cause. But if he had waited much longer, the outcome might have been permanent trouble.

What Causes Ataxia?

Drinking too much frequently culminates in ataxia. We're all familiar with the common scene of the policeman asking a driver to walk a straight line on New Year's Eve. That particular problem in coordination depends on how much alcohol is present in one's system, and gets better as the alcohol wears off. However, an alcoholic may develop permanent damage to some of the balancing mechanisms in the brain, which is why Jay was fortunate to stop drinking when he did.

Alcohol is not the only villain, however. Other causes of ataxia can be much more difficult to treat. For example, loss of coordination may stem from cancer that involves the parts of the brain that control movement. Otherwise, ataxia may come on because the body responds to a cancer as if it is having an allergic reaction, as we discussed in chapter 16, "Cancer and the Brain." The body's immune system makes substances called antibodies to fight the cancer, but these antibodies can affect the brain. When they attack the cerebellum, the result can undermine motor control. Sometimes, when the cancer is found and treated, the ataxia will get better.

Ataxia runs in some families. Researchers have identified a number of different genetic abnormalities that may play a role in this disorder, and they will undoubtedly find many more. The problem usually begins with a gradual loss of coordination, generally when walking or turning. People may have particular difficulty walking at night or walking on uneven ground, such as a lawn or a beach. These problems worsen over the course of years. Other skills such as writing, dressing, or handling cutlery or a cup also erode to the vanishing point.

Regardless of its specific cause, ataxia always attacks the same part of the brain, the cerebellum. Specific nerve cells in the cerebellum die from the toxic effects of alcohol, cancer, or some genetic abnormality. Once these nerve cells in the cerebellum have died, the disease cannot be reversed. That makes early recognition and intervention essential.

Treatment of Ataxia

The treatment of ataxia depends on the cause. If alcohol has caused the ataxia, the individual must stop drinking before permanent damage occurs. If cancer has triggered it, physicians must determine whether the cancer is attacking the brain directly or indirectly, via an overreaction by the immune system. Cancer in the brain can be treated by surgery, radiation, and chemical agents, as we discussed in chapter 10, "How to Keep Your Balance—Literally." When cancer plays an indirect role, treatment must address the underlying cancer and also try to block the immune system's hyperallergic responses. The treatment of hereditary ataxia remains very unsatisfactory. There are no good medications that will decrease the ataxia. In some cases, deep brain stimulation is tried on an experimental basis.

Future Treatments of Ataxia

The understanding of hereditary ataxia is evolving rapidly. In many families it is possible to identify the genetic abnormality involved, and to use this information to determine who is at risk for getting the disease, often many years before symptoms appear. Acquiring this genetic information is an essential step in understanding the disease mechanisms and developing new therapies. If you are part of a family with ataxia, you may want to consider taking part in a clinical study.

OSTEOARTHRITIS OF THE SPINE

Sam, an older man from West Virginia who had spent much of his life working in the coal mines, was finding it progressively difficult to walk. He began to feel very stiff, and he could only shuffle along. He also began having pain when he used his right arm and hand. This was particularly important to him, because he was an expert country fiddler. Besides the pain in his arm, he could no longer handle his bow between a few fingers; he had to try to clamp it with his whole hand, and couldn't control his fingers the way he had before. The fingers of his left hand weren't involved, and he could still whip off a mean "Turkey in the Straw." This was fortunate for us because he used to bring his fiddle when he came up to see us and would entertain patients in the clinic while he was waiting for his appointment.

He first came to see us because another physician had told him that he had ALS, a rapidly progressive degenerative disease, and was going to die. We thought that Sam had an arthritis of the bones of his neck that was gradually getting worse. It was compressing his spinal cord, interfering with the nerve fibers that controlled his legs, and was pressing on the nerves that controlled his right hand. We established that diagnosis with imaging studies of his neck that showed the compression of the spinal cord and nerves, and by electrical studies of nerves and muscles that did not have the abnormal patterns seen in ALS.

Sam had surgery that was successful in relieving his pain and stopping further progression of his problems. His walking became a little bit better, and the use of his right hand improved, although it did not return entirely to normal. Last we heard, he had retired from the coal mines but was playing his fiddle more frequently than ever. Our clinic is a much drearier place without him.

As we discussed in chapter 7, "Pain and Your Brain," the bones of our spine undergo a lot of wear and tear as we get older. When this happens, the bones can press on the nerves exiting from the spinal cord and cause pain or they can compress the spinal cord affecting how signals get from the brain to muscles. The result is that the limbs stiffen, do not move smoothly, and quick movements like those required for turning or balancing are lost, as occurred with Sam.

The compression of the spinal cord usually occurs at two places. In Sam, the major problem was in the neck. In this region, the spinal cord is like a telephone cable, with signals going up and down. Also, nerves exit from the spinal cord at this level to send messages to and from the arms and hands. The other site of problem is the lower spine, causing a narrowing of the space for nerves, a condition called lumbar stenosis. Characteristically, people with this problem are fine while sitting or lying down, but have trouble while on their feet.

In his 80s, Juan still went to his office every day, but walking to lunch became a real ordeal. After only a few steps, his legs would start to tingle and feel weak, as if they were about to buckle. When he sat down, his legs would come back to normal within a minute or two, and he could resume his journey to lunch. Things got so bad that he carefully mapped the strategic places to sit in advance. He encountered similar problems navigating the long concourses to the airline gate in airports. These symptoms also affected his social life. He could no longer stand at a reception or cocktail party for any length of time.

The diagnosis of lumbar stenosis was made with imaging studies of his back. These showed that bony overgrowths in his spine had compressed things so that when he stood up, his lower spinal cord did not get enough blood. The effect was a little like when your legs go to sleep if you sit too long. Surgery gave the nerves more room, and Juan regained considerable function. Walking moderate distances, like going to lunch, ceased to be a problem.

Treatment of Spinal Cord Compression

Even when there is evidence of compression of the spinal cord or the exiting nerves, treatment usually begins with conservative therapy, which includes exercise programs, muscle relaxants, and physical therapy. If this is followed and the symptoms do not decrease or progressively worsen, surgery becomes an option. This surgery removes the bony overgrowths that are pressing on the spinal cord or nerves.

Future Treatment of Spinal Cord Compression

No one knows why the bones around the spine gradually degenerate and press on the spinal cord and nerves. It seems to be more common in people who have had jobs that require a lot of lifting and twisting, like Sam, but it also occurs in people who have spent most of their time sitting at desks, like Juan. Genetic factors may influence who is at risk for this process, but they have not been well worked out. At present nothing can be done to stop the progression of the disorder.

MOTOR NEURON DISEASE OR ALS

The first thing Li, a college professor, noticed was that he started to drool at unexpected times. He began carrying a handkerchief to avoid embarrassment. Within a few weeks he noticed that his voice was changing; he became hoarse and couldn't project his voice as he lectured. Then he encountered difficulty swallowing liquids. Sometimes food would stick in the back of his throat or even go down the wrong way. The first doctor he saw, his primary care physician, couldn't tell what was wrong, but the second, a neurologist, suspected that these were the first symptoms of ALS. The diagnosis was established by studying the electrical activity of his muscles using a technique called electromyography. When muscles are not getting the proper signals from nerves, their electrical properties change. Li's muscles displayed these changes.

Li's disease had announced itself in the muscles involved in swallowing, but in a matter of months it was affecting his hands and legs. The muscles of his hands began to shrink—the medical term is atrophy—so that the bones of his hands became much more prominent. Over larger muscles like his thighs or upper arms, he would notice that his muscles jumped, as if part of a muscle were contracting. This jumping of muscles is called fasciculation.

Within one year of the onset of his symptoms, Li was quite disabled. He had difficulty getting out of a chair, walking, or controlling his hands well enough to pick up a cup. The major problem was in swallowing and talking. He could eat only very slowly, in very small bites. His speech became quite slurred, and only close family members could decipher what he was trying to say. He began using a computer for communication, punching the keys with one finger. His computer was programmed to say or print whole phrases so that his communication could be faster.

Eighteen months after the onset Li was almost bedridden, communicating only by computer. His students came for a tribute to their former teacher. Li had looked forward to this event and had programmed special greetings for each of them, based on their time with him. After that event, he emphasized to his wife and children that he did not want to have any extraordinary measures taken to keep him alive. Consequently he refused to be placed on a respirator as he developed greater problems breathing. Three weeks later he died of pneumonia.

Motor neuron disease is a major cause of progressive difficulty with weakness. The technical name of this disease is amyotrophic lateral sclerosis or ALS. For those of us who remember the old New York Yankees, this disease is, of course, also referred to as Lou Gehrig's disease, honoring their legendary first baseman. The best-selling book *Tuesdays with Morrie* has brought increased attention to this disorder.

In ALS, nerve cells in the spinal cord and the brain that are involved in the control of motor movements progressively deteriorate and die. ALS most often strikes people in their 60s. Some cases start in the 30s and 40s, however, and even more rarely in the 20s. The early symptoms are weakness of the hands and legs, and difficulty swallowing and talking. Many ALS victims become unable to walk and require a wheelchair within two to three years of onset, sometimes even faster. Eventually most people develop weakness of the breathing muscles and need respiratory support with a breathing machine. The disorder is rare, affecting about 25,000 people in the United States.

Physicians generally diagnose ALS by the patterns of weakness found on clinical examination. However, to confirm the diagnosis they must observe/find characteristic changes in the electrical activity of nerves and muscles, as happened with Li. Repeating the electrical studies again after several months can settle any uncertainties in the diagnosis.

What Causes ALS?

In ALS, a specific group of nerve cells dies, in most cases for unknown reasons. The disease affects large nerve cells in the spinal cord that signal to muscles, telling them to move. Polio virus attacks the same nerve cells. This similarity has caused scientists to wonder whether ALS also involves a specific virus or bacteria that infects the nerve cells, like polio, or some toxic substance that damages them. Every few years, scientists report the possibility that an infectious agent, usually a virus, has been found among individuals with ALS. Unfortunately, these findings have not been repeated in other laboratories.

In addition, there sometimes appear to be clusters of the disease, in which a group of individuals who have something in common develop the disease. For example, a group of cases developed among previous members of the San Francisco 49ers professional football team. This made scientists wonder whether exposure to some substance, such as a pesticide spread on the field or steroids used for muscle building, made them sick. However, none of these possible leads panned out.

GENETICS AND ALS

About 15 percent of the time, ALS runs in families, and in some of these families an abnormal form of a gene has been found. This abnormal gene is called super-oxide dismutase or SOD. Mice implanted with this gene develop progressive weakness and loss of nerve cells, and then eventually die. On examination under a microscope, the brains of these mice display the changes seen in ALS. As scientists try to develop methods of treating ALS, they are using these mice to screen for effective medications.

Treatment of ALS

The FDA has approved one drug for treatment of ALS, Riluzole, which somewhat slows the disease's progression. In development are experimental therapies based on substances called trophic factors, which nerve cells require to maintain themselves. Some researchers have focused on a specific factor called brain-derived neurotrophic factor (BDNF), because it is required by the nerve cells in the spinal cord that die in ALS. These substances are still in clinical trials. That means they are available only at selected medical centers, where they are being studied under specific protocols, and are not available to the general public. It is important for ALS patients to be involved in such trials, if possible, for their own benefit and that of future ALS sufferers.

Even in the absence of effective treatments, the advent of computers has immeasurably improved the life of ALS patients. Before computers were widely available, some patients with ALS became unable to communicate once they could no longer speak or write. With computer technology, communication is possible well into the disease. If the patient is able to control the movement of even one finger or toe, he or she can press a computer key. This enables them to write preprogrammed phrases or words to communicate what they are thinking. As movement becomes even more limited, patients use computers with a moving cursor. When the cursor is over a letter that is part of the word the patient wants to write, or over a desired phrase, he or she presses a key. Then the cursor returns to the beginning until the next letter or phrase is selected. Obviously, this makes communication very laborious, but it enables patients to interact with those around them. Since their mental abilities are completely preserved, this technology is a great gift, often enabling them to work in a limited fashion long after they can no longer walk, talk, or eat normally.

Future Treatments of ALS

Medical scientists now have an animal model of ALS for testing medications, and they are evaluating a number of new medications in studies of patients with the disease. In addition to Riluzole, several more drugs should become available within the next few years. There are certain diseases about which it is possible to feel optimisitic. So much has been learned in such a short time that effective treatments seem likely to emerge in the near future. ALS is one of these diseases.

WHAT YOU CAN DO ABOUT SHAKING, WEAKNESS, AND ALS

Shaking and weakness often stem from conditions that can be treated. See your doctor for a thorough investigation. This way you can begin treatment promptly, and a diagnosis of a more serious disease can be confirmed or ruled out. Essential tremor, for example, is treatable in most people, though with different medications than those used for Parkinson's disease, for which it is often mistaken. The movement disorder known as ataxia can often be reversed by cutting out alcohol. On the other hand, ataxia can be a sign of cancer, particularly in individuals who have no family history of the disorder. If you develop these symptoms, you should be evaluated. Similarly, bony disease of the spine can compress nerves and cause muscle weakness. Though treatable with strategies ranging from exercise to surgery, it is sometimes mistaken for amyotrophic lateral sclerosis (ALS), a fatal condition.

If ALS is strongly suspected, however, it's important to seek evaluation at a clinical center with expertise in this disorder; the diagnostic procedure, consisting of electrical studies of the nerves and muscles, can easily be misinterpreted. Besides Riluzole, there are experimental trials with newer agents at several medical centers.

CHAPTER 19

STROKE: THE BRAIN–HEART CONNECTION

In the middle of the Republican National Convention in July 2000, Gerald Ford, the former president of the United States, gave an address to the assembled audience. People were impressed by how fit he looked and how energetic he sounded at the age of 87. The next day, however, several reporters noticed that his speech wasn't normal: he was slurring his words. He understood what everyone was saying to him, and what he was saying made perfect sense. It was just that he couldn't pronounce his words correctly. He also seemed to be having trouble with balance and eventually he needed help walking. Somewhat reluctantly, he went to a nearby hospital, where an imaging study revealed that he had had a small stroke in the back part of his brain—the part of the brain that is involved with balance and coordination of movement. President Ford was placed on blood thinners and gradually began to improve. On the fourth day after the stroke, he left the hospital and returned home.

No two organs in the body interact as closely as do the brain and the heart. The heart pumps oxygen- and nutrient-rich blood to the brain. The brain regulates the pumping, especially its speed, or, in other words, the number of heartbeats per minute. The brain also influences how the heart responds to illness. For example, depression carries a risk of both a greater likelihood of having a heart attack and a poorer survival afterward.

Even with advancing age, the heart and the brain normally work together without a hitch and without our being aware of their inter-actions. An insidious process can silently disrupt their teamwork, however. This process is called arteriosclerotic vascular disease, a hardening and closing of the arteries. It can affect all arteries in the body, but particularly those of the brain and the heart. The end result can be either a heart attack or a stroke, now called a brain attack.

Symptoms of Stroke

The symptoms of stroke depend on what part of the brain is not getting enough blood. A person having a stroke might experience such symptoms as weakness of an arm and hand, sudden loss of vision in one eye, an acute loss of balance, difficulty speaking, or a feeling of numbness over the face. Strokes are usually asymmetrical, that is, they involve only one side of the body.

Strokes can occur in three time frames. In the first sort of time frame a person suffers a brief loss of function called a transient ischemic attack (TIA), sometimes referred to as a mini-stroke. Such episodes rarely last 30 minutes. Although usually not life threatening or permanently damaging in themselves, they indicate that something more severe and long lasting might happen. Many people will have repeated TIAs, sometimes dozens of them. The chance of having a stroke after a series of TIAs is about 25 percent. Thus their recognition and treatment are extremely important.

In the second sort of time frame a stroke has a gradually progressive course. The last time frame is the completed stage of a stroke in which there is persistent change of function, sometimes with only partial recovery.

What Happens during a Stroke?

A stroke occurs when an area of the brain does not receive enough blood. In the brain, the arteries divide a number of times as they extend upward from the carotid artery in the neck, with each branch of an artery supplying blood to its own specific brain territory. When an artery, or a branch of an artery, becomes plugged, the brain cells it is supposed to serve begin to starve for oxygen and nutrients; it's rather like a lawn with a sprinkler system. Specific pipes water specific areas of the lawn. If a pipe gets plugged, its area of the lawn will start to wilt, but it can recover if the flow of water is restored in time. If it is not, then that area of the lawn will turn brown and die. Similarly, if one of the arteries supplying an area of the brain becomes plugged, the nerve cells in that area are initially stunned, and may not work correctly. If blood flow is restored quickly enough, they can recover, but if the lack of blood is too prolonged, they will die.

WHO IS AT RISK FOR A STROKE?

The same factors put one at risk for a heart attack or a stroke. What are these? Age is one. The average age of a first stroke for men is about 70, and for women about 77. But age alone is not usually enough to cause a stroke. The risk of stroke rises as age combines with other predisposing factors such as hypertension (high blood pressure), diabetes, smoking, and high levels of fat and/or cholesterol in the blood. Someone who has high blood pressure is twice as likely to have a stroke as someone the same age who does not. The same is true for diabetes.

Recently another risk factor has been identified, the blood level of a substance called homocysteine, a naturally occurring chemical. If these levels are elevated, some physicians recommend treatment with folic acid and vitamin B_{12} to lower them.

The other reason people have strokes is because a blood clot, or cerebral embolus, plugs a small blood vessel. Small clots flow up toward the brain, carried along by the rapid flow of blood through large arteries. The arteries become smaller and smaller as they branch to supply the substance of the brain. Eventually the clot will be unable to pass through a smaller artery and will plug it.

The heart can easily send clots to the brain. For example, a person who has had a heart attack may have damage in part of the heart muscle. If this section of muscle does not move very well, a clot or clots will form on the wall of the heart. Eventually such a clot can break off and flow through the bloodstream until it gets stuck somewhere. In other cases, bits of material become dislodged from the valves of the heart and work their way through the bloodstream. Clots also form when the heart beats irregularly. Someone whose heart shifts back and forth from a regular to an irregular rhythm faces a particular risk of blood clots being dislodged from the heart and causing trouble elsewhere in the body, including the brain.

The large arteries coming from the heart, the aorta and the carotid arteries, also produce many clots. The two carotid arteries, one on each side of your neck, each divide just under the base of the jaw. (You can feel the pulsations of either or both of the carotid arteries by pressing your fingers gently on your neck in that region.) One branch goes into the head, to supply the brain, and the other branch stays outside to supply the face and scalp. This branching point in the neck, where the artery divides, is where clots of arteriosclerotic material occur. They may build up so much that they may even narrow or close the artery, or bits of this accumulated material can break off and be carried up into the brain.

STROKES ARE DECREASING

Fortunately, fewer and fewer people in the United States are dying from strokes. There are several factors at play. Part of the decrease undoubtedly results from the fact that people are taking better care of themselves.

Another reason strokes are decreasing is that techniques for evaluating the status of arteries and deciding whether they should be cleaned out have improved dramatically. Until very recently the only way to see arteries was by performing a procedure called an arteriogram. In this procedure a dye is injected to outline the arteries and make them more visible by x-ray. This reveals whether an artery has narrowed or contains material that might break off. An advance in MRI technology, called MRI angiography, has made it possible to see the arteries without any injections. With this procedure physicians and surgeons can immediately determine if the arteries are open and carrying blood normally. It is amazing how well the arteries in the neck and the larger arteries in the brain can be seen. It should not be long before a comprehensive physical will include evaluations of the arteries of the heart and brain with these new imaging techniques. MRI is often coupled with a procedure for listening to arteries, called ultrasound. This procedure can show if a vessel is partially clogged, the rate of flow through a vessel, and whether there are small abnormal particles being carried in the flow. Ultrasound can also reveal information about the artery, showing whether it is open or not.

EVALUATION OF STROKE

Clarissa was reading a magazine in her doctor's waiting room when she suddenly realized that something was wrong with her vision. She had the presence of mind to close one eye and then the other, and she noticed that the vision in her right eye was normal. In the left eye, her vision was very blurred, and as she attempted to look at the magazine, she seemed to lose all sight in that eye. She told the receptionist and was immediately examined by the doctor, who looked in her eyes and did not see anything wrong. Within a matter of minutes the vision began to return, and shortly thereafter was entirely normal. The doctor told her to go directly to the hospital's emergency room, but as her vision was now normal and she had plans for the evening, she went home instead. However, that night she had a second episode of exactly the same thing. This frightened her enough to go to the hospital.

When she arrived, the emergency room staff immediately had a CT scan performed, which showed no evidence that Clarissa had any type of bleeding in her brain. She was placed on heparin, a medicine to thin her blood, and watched carefully for a few days. Then her heparin was stopped, and she was switched to one aspirin each day.

The most likely explanation for symptoms like Clarissa's is that some artery is not supplying enough blood to the brain. In her case, it was a small artery supplying the back of her eye, her retina. There are then two questions physicians ask: "What is happening in the brain?" and "What is going on in the circulation of blood from the heart to the brain?"

Brain Imaging

CT scanning machines are accessible in many emergency rooms, making it possible to tell very quickly if the problem is a stroke, a hemorrhage, or a blood clot. It is important to be sure that there is no bleeding in the brain, because one way to treat these warning attacks is to use medicines, called anticoagulants, that will thin the blood, and these medications would make bleeding worse!

Sometimes, a CT image may not show any areas of damage. In these situations, an MRI scan may be revealing, particularly using some of the newer technical tricks, such as Diffusion Weighted Imaging (or DWI), which can show an area of damage within minutes of its onset. Sometimes, doctors also see evidence of old damage in areas of the brain that might not be associated with the recent symptoms. These "silent" areas of damage indicate that the person has been having previous, unrecognized episodes. Usually, however, the abnormalities we see on the images correspond to the person's symptoms.

Evaluating the Heart

The other thing we need to know is the status of the heart. Is it beating at a regular rhythm, or is it beating irregularly? The medical term for an irregularly beating heart is an arrhythmia. The most common arrhythmia is atrial fibrillation. This problem with heart rhythm has been in the news because it has affected both former President Bush and former Senator Bill Bradley. Both these men, like thousands of others, are taking medications to keep their hearts in normal rhythm. This is important because 25 to 30 percent of strokes, particularly in people over 75 years of age, have this form of arrhythmia as a cause. When the heart is beating irregularly, it is more likely that small clots from the heart will break off and go up to the brain.

The presence of an arrhythmia can be detected very quickly with an electrocardiogram, or EKG. Sometimes the heart goes in and out of an irregular rhythm, and may be normal during an examination. Wearing a heart monitor with a continuous recording device for an extended period—perhaps two or more days—will detect and emphasize changes in rhythm.

A rarer cause of clots going to the brain is an abnormal opening between the two sides of the heart. Normally blood returns from the tissues of the body to the heart, is pumped through the lungs where it picks up oxygen, and returns to the heart to be pumped out to the body again. The lungs, besides supplying oxygen, also act as filters, removing small clots that might develop in places like the veins of the legs. However, in some people, an opening in the heart allows some blood to bypass the lungs. When this occurs, clots that should have been filtered out can go to the brain. This condition is diagnosed by introducing small bubbles of gas into the heart and seeing where they go. The abnormal opening can be closed surgically with a patch or by a form of cardiac catheterization.

TREATMENT OF STROKE

Treatment of TIAs

Clarissa had a TIA. The most likely cause of Clarissa's TIA is that a small clot broke off from her heart or a carotid artery and went up to the artery to her eye. The goal of treatment is to keep other clots from doing the same thing or going to other arteries supplying the brain. The first line of defense is a very simple compound, plain old aspirin. One each day is enough! Aspirin works by keeping a component of blood, platelets, from clumping together. The clumping together of platelets is an essential step in the formation of clots. An individual who takes aspirin after a TIA is only two-thirds as likely to have stroke as one who does not. There are some people who cannot take aspirin, usually because it upsets their stomach. For them, "antiplatelet" compounds such as Ticlopidine and Clopidogrel can substitute. But some people continue to have TIA's despite these antiplatelet medications. What to do then?

The next step up in preventing further problems is to thin the blood more aggressively. There are two types of compounds: Heparin, used on a short-term basis and usually given by injection, and Warfarin, or Coumadin, taken in pill form and used on a longer term basis. Cardiologists prescribe these blood thinners to prevent problems with heart attacks, as well as to prevent strokes in people who have irregular beating of the heart or who have had artificial heart valves implanted. Both compounds interfere with blood clotting mechanisms, preventing the formation of clots.

Thinning of the blood can significantly reduce the risk of stroke, particularly for people with a heart arrhythmia. Those taking Warfarin have only one-third the number of strokes as those who do not. The downside is that a person using these blood-thinners for long periods of time might have a serious bleeding problem after a fall or accident.

Clarissa had no further episodes for about six months. Then she began having a different kind of problem—brief episodes of weakness of the right arm. Taking aspirin had no effect on the new problem, and she was switched to Coumadin. When the episodes of weakness in her arm continued, she had an arteriogram. This revealed over a 70 percent narrowing of her left carotid artery, the artery that supplies blood to her left eye and the left side of her brain. However, the left side of the brain controls the movements of the right side of her body—hence the weakness of her right side. Clarissa had surgery to remove the plaque from inside the artery, and she is now doing well, taking one aspirin per day with no further attacks.

Treatment of Blocked Arteries

The build-up of plaque in an artery results in the interior bore of the passageway becoming smaller and smaller, resulting in the narrowing known as stenosis; eventually, the artery can become completely plugged. Thus, the narrowing of the carotid artery is called carotid artery stenosis. When a carotid artery, one of the four major arteries supplying the brain, is found to be clogged or thought to be the source for clots to the brain, surgery to open the artery may be required. This surgery is called carotid artery endarterectomy. Two groups of people are candidates for this procedure: One group consists of those who have carotid artery stenosis, but have never had any associated symptoms. In the past, these people were usually detected because a physician heard a noise when listening over the neck with a stethoscope. As MRI angiography and ultrasound are used more frequently, detection of these partially closed arteries is becoming more common, even in people with no associated symptoms. The the current medical consensus is that surgery should not be performed unless narrowing of the artery is so severe that less than 30 percent of it remains open.

The other group considered for surgery consists of those who have symptoms, such as repeated TIA's, originating from the side of the brain that receives its blood supply from the partially plugged artery. Physicians pay particular attention to those who are having repeated TIA's despite the use of aspirin or more stringent blood thinners (such as Clarissa). In this group, narrowing to less than 30 percent of the normal diameter of the artery is an indication for surgery. Under these prerequisites, those with surgery have one-third fewer strokes than those who are treated only with aspirin.

Many people who have carotid artery surgery are elderly and have significant medical problems related to other organs, particularly the heart. Therefore, the best results are obtained when treatment is given by teams of neurologists and vascular surgeons or neurosurgeons. The team should be organized so that it performs a significant number of these procedures per year, because, as the saying goes, practice makes perfect, or as nearly so as is humanly possible. For these sorts of surgeries, a team needs to work together regularly to stay sharp. After surgery, the artery may close up again. The status of the artery can be determined by repeating ultrasound tests or MRI angiography. Both of these tests are totally noninvasive; all the person has to do is lie there, while the arteries are examined by sound waves (in the case of ultrasound) or changes in magnetic signal (in the case of MRI). The most likely time for the artery to become closed up again is in the first year, and that happens to about 10 percent of the people who have this operation. After that the incidence of reclosure falls off to 3 percent in the second year and 2 percent in the third. The long-term risk of reclosure is about 1 percent per year. That means that 99 of 100 people will not require repeat surgery if they make it through the first three years.

What Blood Is Carrying to Your Brain

The blood supply to the brain carries essential nutrients, but most importantly oxygen. The cells of your brain, like all the other cells in your body, require a continuous supply of oxygen to function. Oxygen, a component of the air you breathe, is absorbed through your lungs into the blood where it then attaches to a component of red blood cells, hemoglobin. These oxygen-carrying red blood cells circulate from the lungs to your heart and then are pumped out to the tissues of the body. The oxygen then leaves the red blood cells and seeps into the cells of the tissues. In the cells, small packets of enzymes—called mitochondria—concentrate oxygen and use it to burn up glucose to create the energy cells need to function. In this process, the brain does not differ from other organs and body tissues except that brain cells are unusually susceptible to the lack of oxygen. Thus, if for some reason, there is not enough oxygen in the blood, such as after a heart attack and cardiac arrest, the brain suffers disproportionately and is the limiting factor in whether or not a person returns to normal.

Nothing can substitute for oxygen, and there is no such thing as a purified source. When someone has difficulty breathing, he or she often receives extra oxygen through a mask or a tube. In some unusual circumstances it is possible to force extra oxygen into tissues by putting a person in a high-pressure chamber for brief periods of time, for instance, people who get the "bends" from diving too deeply in the water for too long, burn victims, and people whose skin has been damaged by radiation. Attempts have been made to use high-pressure treatments to reverse strokes or other brain damage, but without success.

How long the nerve cells can survive after the blood supply is interrupted depends on several factors, primarily the body temperature. At the normal body temperature (98°F or 37°C) the nerve cells start to die within a few minutes. The cooler one is, the longer the interval one can go without damage. That is why surgeons perform some operations on the brain with the body and brain cooled down to 30°C, or even lower. This helps protect the brain from possible periods of lack of blood flow. It also explains occasional stories in the media about people who survived near-drowning without brain damage because they were in nearly ice-cold water.

Progressive Strokes

Many strokes do not just suddenly occur. There may be a "stuttering" onset with intermittent symptoms over several hours, or even a day or two.

Marianna, a college teacher in her 60s, was leading a discussion of American History, when she suddenly couldn't speak clearly. When she said the name "Adams," it sounded more like "Dums." She also had a slight headache and felt a little dizzy. She waited, tried to speak again in a minute or so, and then she seemed all right. At lunch the same thing happened again, only this time she also had trouble using her right hand to hold her coffee cup. By now quite frightened, she called her son, who had difficulty understanding her on the telephone. He came and took her to the hospital. By the time she was examined, several hours after the start of her problems, she had difficulty using her right arm and leg.

Evaluation of Progressive Strokes

Time is of the essence in evaluating and treating people such as Marianna. The evaluation is very similar to those used with TIA's. Doctors ask the same questions—"What's the status of the brain and what's the status of the blood vessels and heart?"—but here the emphasis is different. Things are going sour and something has to be done fast.

Treatment of Progressive Strokes

One of the reasons to call a stroke a "brain attack" is to change people's thinking. The "Nothing can be done, so why hurry" attitude that was once prevalent in neurology has disappeared. Cardiologists have become very aggressive in how they treat patients with heart attacks. They quickly use agents that will unplug the coronary arteries to the heart. Neurologists are learning from our heart specialist colleagues, and are now using agents that will open up plugged arteries. This approach to treatment requires that a person who has a stroke begin receiving treatment very quickly, preferably within three hours of the onset of the stroke. The first step is an immediate imaging study to determine that the stroke is not due to a hemorrhage. At the same time, an MRI angiography can show which vessel is plugged. At this point, the strategy is a little like trying to unblock the pipe in your sink with Drano. The medicine that unplugs arteries by dissolving clots is called tPA (short for tissue-type plasminogen activator). It is given by injection right in the emergency room. When this unplugging of an artery works, the results can be spectacularly successful. The disabilities from the stroke can disappear immediately.

The major complication is that some people may have a problem with bleeding in the brain after this treatment. People with high blood pressure seem to be susceptible to this complication. A newer experimental approach is to thread a small tube, called a catheter, into the blocked artery, and to deliver the unblocking agent right into the artery. This new experimental method may use a different form of "Drano" called urokinase. It may be the approach of the future, particularly for people who are delayed in receiving treatment until six to seven hours after the onset of the stroke. These newer approaches require teams of neurologists and specially trained radiologists who are ready to move fast. It is unlikely that this technology will be available at local hospitals. Instead, stroke victims will be brought to "brain attack centers," which are forming in many large hospitals, in the same way that people with acute trauma, such as head injuries, are rushed to regional trauma centers.

A second treatment is to use blood thinners very aggressively—giving injections of heparin for several days, even a week or two, then switching to the longer-acting blood thinner, Warfarin (also known as Coumadin), on which the patient can stay for months.

Marianna was rushed to the neuroradiology suite for an MRI, which showed no bleeding. An arteriogram showed a blockage in a branch of a major artery in the left side of her brain. Guided by an x-ray machine, a surgeon threaded a catheter up that artery. Then the chemical tPA was injected through the catheter to break up the material that was clogging the artery. While she was on the x-ray table, Marianna's speech began to return and the use of her right arm improved. She left the hospital a few days later, not entirely back to normal, but much better. She is still taking Coumadin as a blood thinner, but otherwise doing well. She plans to return to her teaching in the fall.

STROKE AND REHABILITATION

Not all strokes get better. Anxiety about this raises many questions for patients and their families. Who will recover? Can the outcome be predicted? What is the role of physical therapy and speech therapy? Can medications aid recovery?

One way of addressing these issues is to see what happens to stroke patients after they leave the hospital. Of stroke victims who require hospitalization, about 50 percent go home and 20 percent die in the hospital. Of the remaining 30 percent, about half go to nursing homes and half to rehabilitation units. Rehabilitation units are primarily for those who were independent before their strokes, have normal cognitive function, (think clearly), have a supportive environment, and a home to go to after discharge. A person in rehabilitation also has to be able to tolerate up to three to four hours of various forms of therapy each day. Finally, in today's climate, one of the factors that determine whether a person receives rehabilitation after acute hospitalization is available insurance.

Recovery of Walking after Stroke

At the time of admission to a general rehabilitation hospital for treatment of problems with walking, about 50 percent of the patients cannot walk at all, about 10 percent can walk only with assistance, and the remaining 40 percent do not walk normally but can walk without help. Recovery, if it occurs, is likely to come within the first three months after the stroke. If there is no improvement after six months, it is unlikely that further physical therapy will be of benefit. The good news is that after about one month of rehabilitation, two-thirds of the patients are walking independently. The recovered walking may be slow, one-half the normal speed, but people are getting around on their own.

Recovery of Use of the Hand after Stroke

As with walking, the degree of recovery depends on the severity of the initial handicap. For those with mild problems, 80 percent recover good use of the hand within 6 weeks. In contrast, for those with a severe disability, only 20 percent recover by 12 weeks. Some continued partial recovery could occur up to a year or more after the stroke.

Language Recovery after Stroke

About one-third of people with strokes have a problem, called an aphasia, in understanding or expressing language. Among these patients, about one-half will have improved by 12 weeks after a stroke. Those who recover start early, within days. Most recovery occurs by three months, but there may be some further improvement, particularly in understanding. Some aspects of language, especially comprehension, can continue to recover for several years.

If possible, a person should be evaluated by a speech therapist soon after the stroke, so that the best approach to therapy can be planned. The actual therapy can be carried out by an amateur, such as a spouse or other family member, but this person will need some training and continuing guidance by a speech therapist.

What Determines Recovery of Language Problems Due to Stroke?

There are several factors that influence recovery, including the amount of the brain that has been damaged, the location of the damage, and the person's age (in general, older people do not do as well as younger people). However, there is great variation among individuals. Often a person who seemed a poor candidate for improvement does remarkably well. Consequently all stroke victims should receive speech therapy, no matter how severe the language deficit. If there is no progress after a few months, then the therapy will likely not be of help. Interestingly, left-handers seem to do better than right-handers. That may be because, in left-handers, language may be represented in both sides of the brain, not just primarily on the left (as it is in right-handers).

If speech therapy is not started immediately, it is still worth a try; it can be beneficial even weeks after the stroke.

Evaluation for Rehabilitation

The problems after a stroke can be quite different, depending on both the size and location of the injury. There is no such thing as a universal stroke rehabilitation program; rehabilitation must be tailored to an individual's deficits and needs.

The first step is careful evaluation of the nature of the stroke and the subsequent functional deficit. This evaluation can provide the basis for predicting a likely outcome. But only in a rough way; much remains unknown about why one person improves and another does not.

There are many schools of thought about forms of rehabilitation. Our view is that there is little basis for favoring one particular method. Different individuals will benefit from different approaches.

Computer-based training programs offer many possibilities for reha-bilitation. For example, to aid recovery of the arm, a person might combine physical therapy with a robotic training program. In this program, moving a lever moves objects displayed on a screen. This approach combines aspects of motor learning, motor movement, and visual feedback of what is happening. Whatever form of therapy is used, it should be started early.

A new approach to therapy, particularly to promote use of a weak arm and/or hand, is to restrain the use of the normal, unaffected limb. Usually the normal limb is placed in a sling, and intensive motor ther-apy is applied to the involved side for a period of two to three weeks. For some patients, particularly those with less severe weakness, this form of therapy can be of help.

A crucial question with rehabilitation therapy is when to stop. As mentioned above, for most deficits, recovery occurs within the first three months. However, some of the robotic-based programs may be useful even in those with delayed recovery. There is little evidence that con-ventional therapy for motor problems aids recovery after six months.

Changes in Behavior after Stroke

In addition to the problems with movement and speech, a variety of behavioral changes may occur after stroke.

Depression after Stroke

Anyone who has a stroke, or experiences some other kind of medical catastrophe, is likely to feel a range of emotions such as grief, anger, fear, and discouragement. These reactions are quite normal. But some kinds of mood disturbances are not purely psychological reactions to illness and disability; they are often deficits in themselves, resulting from damage to the neural circuitry underlying the emotions. For example, about 20 percent of people will have severe depression after a stroke, and another 20 percent will have milder forms of depression. Depression hampers recovery after stroke and is also associated with a decreased rate of survival. Thus it is important to recognize and to treat depression, keeping in mind that it can be a form of stroke-induced damage like speech or motor disturbance, not a mere case of the blues that the patient should be exhorted to "snap out of."

When someone is going along in life perfectly normally and then, out of the blue, loses a major area of functioning, it is not surprising that he or she becomes depressed. What is surprising is that not all strokes produce depression in the same way. Those strokes involving the front part of the brain, particularly the left frontal lobe (an area involved in planning of actions, planning of speech, and the output of speech), are more likely to result in depression in the first few months after a stroke. When strokes occur in the right hemisphere, depression is more likely to come on later.

The wife of a colleague, a woman in her 70s, had a stroke that involved the front part of the left side of her brain. Initially, she had difficulty expressing herself and using her right hand. She made a significant recovery over the first three months, and by that time could write, somewhat slowly, and could speak, even converse on the telephone. She was really doing very well, but she did not think so. She went into a shell, refusing to go out of the house and sometimes spending the entire day in bed. It took some time to recognize that this woman was severely depressed. With proper antidepressant medications, in this case Prozac, she made a seemingly miraculous recovery. Much of her functional disability was not from her stroke, but from her depression.

The symptoms of post-stroke depression are the same as those that plague people who have depression for other reasons. Feelings of sadness, anxiety, inability to concentrate, difficulty sleeping with early morning awakening, and morbid thoughts, including thoughts of death, characterize depression in either case. Less commonly, people may become paranoid, accusing their caregivers of stealing from them or trying to poison them. Depression after a stroke will usually respond to treatment, but it may take as long as 12 weeks before the full beneficial effects are evident. After that, treatment has to be continued for months. It may make a difference what antidepressant medications are used. The older drug Nortryptilene appears to be more effective than the newer SSRI drugs (which we discussed in chapter 4, "Managing Stress").

Difficulty Controlling Emotions after Stroke

"Emotional liability," or difficulty controlling emotions, is a common problem after stroke. Sometimes it is associated with depression, at other times it occurs independently.

Steve had what seemed to be a rather minor stroke. For a few weeks he had difficulty speaking, particularly when he got tired. What really bothered him, and his family, was uncontrollable crying, which happened in our office several times in the space of 30 minutes. While asking about his family, we asked whether his parents were still alive. As he answered the question tears came to his eyes and he started to quietly cry. He became quite embarrassed and kept saying "this is not me." Even though we did not think Steve was depressed, his crying did get better with a low dose of an antidepressant.

As with depression, it's important to remember that the condition results from a specific pattern of damage to the brain—most likely the circuitry involved in stopping inappropriate behavior—and does not represent a lack of willpower on the part of the patient.

Hemorrhage in the Brain

Thelma, an elderly woman, came into the emergency room complaining of the sudden onset of the worst headache she had ever had in her life. The emergency room physician was busy and thought maybe she just had the flu. He gave her some pain medicine and told her to lie down, that he would check on her again. When he came back to see her a few minutes later, she was confused; the doctor had trouble getting her attention. When she spoke she again complained of a very severe headache. She said her neck was stiff and the bright lights hurt her eyes. It was clear that something was terribly wrong and that her condition was becoming worse. She was rushed to the brain imaging suite, and a CT scan indicated that she had blood surrounding her brain. An arteriogram, the injection of dye into the arteries, was performed and indicated that a small outpouching on an artery in her brain, an aneurysm, had leaked. She was taken immediately to the operating room. With the assistance of an operating microscope, surgeons placed a small clip on the aneurysm to prevent any further bleeding. She had a few rocky days in the intensive care unit, but gradually made a complete recovery. This all happened about three years ago, and she has been perfectly fine ever since.

Most strokes are caused by the closing up of an artery, as we have described above. However, there is another cause which is much more dramatic and fortunately less common. This form of stroke is the disruption of the brain that occurs when there is sudden bleeding into the brain.

What Causes Bleeding inside the Head?

When blood leaks out of blood vessels it irritates the coverings of the brain. A stiff neck and severe headache are the tip-off that such an event has occurred. An artery, as with Thelma, may be abnormal. It may have the thinning or outpouching of the wall, like a weak spot in a garden hose, which we call an aneurysm. When the pressure in the hose goes up, water will squirt out through the leak. Due to the pressure in a brain artery, an aneurysm can suddenly leak, allowing blood to escape.

It is not clear why aneurysms occur. If one person in a family has an aneurysm, others in the family are likelier to do so as well, in comparison to the population as a whole, but no clear-cut patterns of heredity have emerged. They are increasingly common with age, and more common in women than men.

The advances in imaging of the brain have created a new dilemma. When studying the brain for some other problem, doctors may detect aneurysms that have never caused any symptoms. Should they be treated? The consensus is to leave these outpouchings alone unless they are quite large. They can easily be monitored by repeated imaging every 6 to 12 months. If they are getting bigger, then surgery may be necessary.

A second, less common cause of bleeding is a congenital abnormality in the development of blood vessels in the brain, resulting in a tangle of abnormal vessels called vascular malformations. When these malformations cause trouble they do not suddenly break but instead leak small amounts of blood into the brain. The symptoms are much less severe and not nearly as life-threatening as with an aneurysm. An MRI may find these malformations. They are often totally nonsymptomatic, and if this is the case, they are usually best left alone.

High blood pressure can also cause a blood vessel to "blow." Bleeding in the brain as a result of high blood pressure usually occurs without warning. The symptoms depend on where in the brain the bleeding occurs. Unlike that from aneurysms, the bleeding from high blood pressure is more likely to be deep inside the brain, and it is often fatal. Prevention lies in detecting high blood pressure and keeping it under control.

The Diagnosis of Bleeding in the Brain

A headache like Thelma's, which comes out of the blue and is so severe that it may feel more painful than any previous headache a person has had, often indicates bleeding in or around the brain. Before the days of modern brain imaging, doctors had to perform a procedure called a lumbar puncture or spinal tap, to look for evidence of blood seeping down the spinal cord from the brain. Now a CT scan, often done right in the emergency room, can provide the same information quickly without the bother and risk of an invasive procedure. If there is bleeding, the next question is where it came from. Sometimes the imaging study will show this. It may reveal a collection of blood deep within the brain, or a tangle of abnormal blood vessels. If imaging studies do not show where the blood came from, an arteriogram can outline the brain's blood vessels. This will highlight any aneurysm or vascular malformation.

Treatment for Bleeding in the Brain

Surgery is the first line of therapy for bleeding in the brain. The goal of such surgery depends on the nature of the problem. If there is an aneurysm, the surgeon tries to remove it, usually by putting a clip across the outpouching of the blood vessel. If there is a malformation of the vessels, the surgeon will try to remove that. If there is a collection of blood deep within the brain, the surgeon will try to drain the blood away. Today surgeons operate on many patients they would not have dared to touch in the past. Highly specific angiography, which precisely defines the affected blood vessels, and the operating microscope, which provides necessary magnification, make this high-risk microsurgery feasible. But much depends on the surgeon's skill. Imagine using very delicate instruments to sew together tiny wire filaments, which are jumping around as the heart beats, and you can visualize the problem. This is becoming a very highly specialized area of neurosurgery. If your surgeon does not operate on aneurysms or blood vessels in the brain regularly, try to find someone who does.

Besides advances in surgical technique, new ways to treat the effects of blood on the arteries of the brain have emerged. When blood escapes from leaky blood vessels, it irritates the intact vessels and causes them to clamp down, or constrict. This constriction limits the supply of blood to those areas of the brain, making matters even worse. Recently drugs that affect how calcium is taken up by blood vessels have been found to block the constriction of these vessels. These drugs can help patients with bleeding in the brain both before and after surgery.

RESEARCH IN STROKES

Thinking about the prevention and treatment of patients with strokes has undergone remarkable revision in just the last few years. Many years ago, a stroke was considered almost an expected part of aging. Very little thought was given to preventing strokes or to protecting the injured brain. It was as if strokes were "acts of God" to be met with passive acceptance. We predict that there will be further advances in prevention and in attempts to limit damage during the acute phase of the stroke and to promote recovery, the area most in need of improvement. In short, a very passive area of medicine has now become very active.

Prevention of Strokes

The prevention of strokes goes hand in hand with the prevention of diseases of blood vessels of the heart. Good nutrition, healthy exercise, and giving up smoking are all important factors. In addition, the status of arteries, both those of the heart and those supplying the brain, can now be monitored by new imaging techniques. If a carotid artery is gradually narrowing because of arteriosclerotic disease, then prophylactic surgery can be done. Some of the advances in surgery may make this a much simpler procedure than at present.

Treatment of Strokes

Two advances in brain imaging will help revolutionize the treatment of strokes. The first, called diffusion weighted imaging, or DWI, shows what part of the brain, if any, has been irreversibly damaged. The other, called magnetic resonance perfusion imaging, or MRPI, measures whether the arteries to the brain are delivering as much blood as they should. In combination, these two new techniques can reveal not only what has actually happened to the brain but also whether there is a reasonable chance that increasing the flow of the blood to the brain will be of any benefit.

We recently had the opportunity to use these two new imaging techniques in experimental treatment of several patients who had narrowing of a carotid artery in the neck as well as strokes that damaged language functions such as naming objects. Imaging studies four to five days after the stroke indicated that there had been very little irreversible damage to the brain, as indicated by DWI, but that the language areas of the brain were not getting enough blood, as indicated by MRPI. Going on the assumption that these parts of the brain which were poorly supplied with blood, but not yet damaged, could still be salvageable, physicians were very aggressive in our treatments, either opening up the narrowed artery surgically, or dramatically increasing the individual's blood pressure to push more blood into the brain. Not only did the language problems get much better but also the repeated imaging studies showed no more brain damage and much better perfusion of the areas of the brain previously undersupplied with blood. These still experimental techniques will surely become part of the standard management of stroke patients in the future.

Protecting Brain Cells after Stroke

Another approach to the treatment of an acute stroke is to use agents that will prevent damage to nerve cells. This is the same strategy that one uses to try and protect the brain after it has suffered from lack of oxygen. When a nerve cell is injured, it releases its contents including the amino acid, glutamate, into the surrounding environment. Glutamate normally serves as a neurotransmitter, one of the substances that nerve cells use to communicate with one another. In normal amounts, glutamate is excitatory, that is, it has a positive effect on another cell. However, too much glutamate leads to the death of the surrounding nerve cells. Thus, the release of glutamate from a damaged nerve cell leads to death of the surrounding nerve cells, essentially expanding the area of dysfunction. There are a variety of substances being tried in animal models of stroke to see if they will block this damage by glutamate.

Predicting Outcomes after Stroke

After the stroke that incapacitated her right hand, Clarissa got better over the next few hours. Another patient with the identical circumstances might have no improvement even after one year. At present no one can predict which patients will recover and which will not. Early improvement of function is a good omen for eventual recovery. What the brain is actually doing during this recovery phase is not clear. Is the damaged area having a return of function? Do other parts of the brain take over these missing functions? The use of imaging techniques that measure the function of the brain may answer these questions. An active area of research is the development and evaluation of medications that can promote recovery after a stroke. Trials are now going on to see if these medications can speed the process of recovery. Some of them will be used immediately after a stroke has occurred to prevent any further damage to the brain. Others will be used during the recovery process. Both types of drugs have been shown to be effective in animal experiments, and will be tried in people in the near future.

HEART SURGERY AND THE BRAIN

For people with chest pain from their heart, so-called angina, the first line of treatment is medication. Many such people continue to have chest pain despite medication, however, particularly when they exert themselves. Coronary artery bypass grafting, often referred to as CABG, may help these people. In this procedure, the person is placed on a pump that replaces the heart's actions, the heart is stopped, and grafts are made from veins from the leg and placed so that they carry blood around the blocked blood vessels in the heart. For those with severe angina, CABG can effectively relieve the symptoms. Over 500,000 people in the United States have this procedure done each year.

In some people, effects on the brain may somewhat offset the relief of heart symptoms. The most feared complication is a stroke during surgery. This occurs less than 5 percent of the time but is more frequent in older people with diabetes, high blood pressure, or evidence of previous strokes. In these high-risk patients, many surgeons modify how they do the procedure.

The other complication relates to how well a person can think and function intellectually. After surgery many people say that they are "not quite the same." This complaint usually refers to memory problems, an inability to take in new information and use it properly that usually lasts a few months and then gradually gets better. Some people, however, have longer-term difficulty with planning and with figuring out how to solve problems. For example, a lawyer can no longer handle complex cases. A chess player can no longer practice playing against the computer because he has trouble planning more than three or four moves ahead. An accomplished scientist has to be very careful when he goes to an out-of-town meeting, because he gets lost trying to find his way from his hotel to the meeting center, which may be only a few blocks away. These postoperative symptoms may persist for months, if not years.

Another common complaint by both the person who has had surgery and his or her family and associates, is a change in personality. Some get depressed; others are more irritable and less able to withstand frustration.

The mechanism of these problems is not entirely clear. They are probably related to small bits of material from the diseased blood vessels that go up into the brain at the time of surgery. Changes in surgical technique, such as heart surgery without the bypass pump, may decrease the likelihood of these longer-term problems.

PERSONALITY AND BEHAVIOR AND THE HEART

Up until now, we have been exploring the effect of the heart on the brain. What about the reverse, the effect of the brain on the heart? Do brain-centered factors like personality or stress alter how one responds to diseases of the heart?

Personality and the Heart

Popular opinion holds that hard-driving, aggressive "Type A" personalities are more likely to have heart disease and heart attacks. However, the evidence for this is rather weak. There is evidence that a Type A person is likely to do better after a heart attack, perhaps because Type As are more motivated to participate in cardiac rehabilitation and lifestyle modification programs.

Stress and Anxiety and the Heart

Related to the issue of personality type is the issue of stress and anxiety and how people handle these factors in their lives. The bottom line in this area is that stress hurts the heart, particularly if the heart is not normal. Repeated studies have shown higher rates of repeat heart attacks and even death in those with high levels of stress and anxiety after a heart attack. The jury is out on whether programs designed to relieve stress make a difference in these poorer outcomes.

Depression and the Heart

A colleague of ours started a study of her medical school classmates over 50 years ago. She sent out a health questionnaire every year to three successive classes from medical school, and it became a matter of pride for each class to respond as completely as possible. Over 90 percent participated. This study showed that among physicians who reported experiencing or being treated for depression, the numbers of heart attacks were increased, strongly suggesting that depression predisposed to disease of the arteries of the heart.

Depression also influences how one does after a heart attack. If a person is significantly depressed after a heart attack, the chance of dying within the first 6 months is 4 times higher, and in the first 18 months, 8 times higher, than for those who are not depressed.

The obvious question is, "Why don't people just treat the depression and be done with it?" That turns out not to be so easy in people with heart disease. Some of the drugs used for depression, such as Elavil, are bad for the heart. They can cause irregular rhythms and low blood pressure. Similarly, electroconvulsive treatments (ECT) affect heart function unless used very carefully. There is hope that the newer drugs for depression, the selective serotonin reuptake inhibitors (the SSRI's) like Prozac and Paxil, will be safer. That leaves psychological therapy to relieve stress and depression. This can work, and many programs include psychological support therapy as part of cardiac rehabilitation.

The interaction of stress and mood with response to heart illness has been sadly neglected until quite recently. Much of the medical literature about treating your heart does not even mention it. That should and will change. Depression and the handling of stress are two of the most powerful factors in determining the outcome after a heart attack. More important, they are factors that a person can do something about. You can't change your genetic makeup or reverse preexisting heart disease, or change your emotional responses like flipping a switch. But you can get treatment for serious mood disorders and shore up your defenses against stress, ensuring that emotions don't add to the toll of heart disease.

WHAT YOU CAN DO ABOUT STROKE: GET HELP FAST

Beginning in the mid-1990s, treatments for stroke became available for the first time, beginning a nationwide effort to view stroke as a medical emergency similar to a heart attack. These medications are called acute treatments, meaning they must be given very soon after the stroke occurs, preferably within three hours. It's crucial to know the warning signs of stroke. According to the American Stroke Association, these signs include:

- Sudden numbness or weakness of the face, arm, or leg, especially on one side of the body
- Sudden confusion, trouble speaking or understanding
- Sudden trouble seeing in one or both eyes
- Sudden trouble walking, dizziness, loss of balance or coordination
- Sudden, severe headache with no known cause

Have the family learn the warning signs as well, perhaps putting up a list wherever you post other first aid and emergency instructions for family members. And call 911 or have someone drive you to the emergency room; don't try to drive yourself.

CHAPTER 20

TAKING CHARGE OF YOUR BRAIN

Change is often most closely associated with youth, not age. Many people consider the milestones of youth—learning to walk, learning to read, graduation, careers, marriage, and children—to be more appealing. But the second half of life is a time of many changes as well. The brain holds some happy surprises for those on the way to their second half: a deeper, richer way with words and a more extensive vocabulary; an ability to learn that's just as complete as in the younger days, though not as quick; the gift of experience, versus the speed of youth, in decision-making and judgment; the ability to appreciate the richness of life. Nevertheless, there are changes that are unwished for. Some are a nuisance—not being able to move as quickly, hear as well, or remember names. Others are associated with more serious problems that need to recognized and treated. As you navigate through the changes of the second half, we hope this book will serve as an adequate map. But here are some compass headings that will keep you in the right direction, maintaining those positive powers of the ever-better brain and moving the odds always more in your favor if undesired problems come along.

In chapter 1, "Maintaining Your Memory," we talked about a study in which our research group studied 1,200 individuals between the ages of 70 and 80 and performing in the top third of the population of this age group. We kept track of these individuals for the next 10 years. Some people at the end of that time had preserved excellent mental functioning, while others had not. We were struck by the fact that those who preserved their mental functions were doing three things the others were not:

1. They were more physically active.
2. They were more mentally active.

3. They maintained a sense of effectiveness in the world around them, meaning that they continued to maintain a sense of control over their lives, felt that they were contributing to their family or to society, and generally felt good about themselves, too.

Learning from that study, we have some suggestions for you.

EXERCISE

Again and again we have emphasized the benefits of physical activity. At the very least, moderate exercise will ameliorate the common problems that people have as they get older, such as weakness, stiffness of the joints, and problems with balance. Exercise also maintains cardiovascular fitness and lung function and helps keep weight under control.

But the pluses go beyond physical fitness; research shows that exercise helps to sharpen cognitive skills, lift depression, and ward off the changes in memory associated with age. This is particularly true for older women where studies suggest that exercise is associated with lower incidences of dementia, even of Alzheimer's disease. The question is, why? To answer that we have to turn to studies with laboratory animals, such as the rat. Human beings are not rats, of course, but there's nothing to lose, and much to gain, from assuming that the same principles will apply.

When rats are given free access to an exercise wheel, the brain's memory nexus, the hippocampus, is larger; these rats also perform better in mazes that test their memories. Other studies in rats show that unlimited opportunity to exercise increases levels of two growth factors, substances produced in the brain that nourish nerve cells and encourage them to grow and proliferate. This increase is most noticeable in the hippocampus. Interestingly, one of these growth factors (called brain-derived neurotrophic factor or BDNF) also increases in response to antidepressant drugs. So by sticking to a regular program of moderate exercise you may be stimulating your brain's natural antidepressant. This is important, because depression is often the associated with many of the problems of aging. The other growth factor that surges during exercise is nerve growth factor (NGF), also prominent in the hippocampus. Based on experiments in which animals get transplants of NGF-producing cells, there's evidence that this growth can reverse age-related memory impairment, at least in rats; other researchers have used NGF treatments to prevent memory decline in older rats. If exercise is so good for a rat's brain, why not for yours as well?

Exercise doesn't have to be brutal. Walking or swimming are excellent, as is lifting light weights at home or riding a stationary bicycle. A simple program may include sit-ups with the knees bent and riding a stationary bike for 15 to 20 minutes each morning. When the weather permits, walk or ride your bike two or three times each week. You'll find that even these simple exercises improve your balance and energy level and will generally make you feel better during the day.

A final note about exercise: If you've never exercised before, it's never too late to start. In a study of over 72,000 women aged 40 to 65, the simple exercise of walking proved to be as effective in preventing heart disease as more strenuous workouts—even if the women had only begun their exercise programs when the study began!

BE MENTALLY ACTIVE

There's good reason to believe that the phrase "Use it or lose it" applies to the brain. What is even better is that you don't have to do anything so very special to keep your mind in shape. In the study mentioned above, those who maintained their mental abilities kept their minds active through such stimulating activities as reading books, doing crossword puzzles, using a computer, and going to lectures or concerts. It is worth noting that the group better at maintaining their mental abilities was less likely to spend time in the passive mode of watching television.

Going back to the rat studies, it's been shown that an enriched environment (one that includes exercise, toys, mirrors, tunnels, and interaction with other rats) strengthens connections between nerve cells in the hippocampus and even increases the rate at which new cells are born (a process known as neurogenesis). Other animal studies show that a stimulus repeated many times (what humans would call rehearsal) results in more synapses, or points of connection, between nerve cells. The more synapses, the more thoroughly a memory is entrenched.

Repetition isn't the only way to reinforce memory; the neurotransmitters called forth during intense emotion can do it as well, and so can plain old concentration. Many older people underutilize their ability to concentrate on the thing they are trying to remember. It isn't that they can't focus attention, but that they don't seem to remember that learning takes work. Just by concentrating on what you want to remember, your memory will improve dramatically.

Some specific strategies have been proven to help. The hippocampus, for example, is the center of both directional and contextual memory—supplying the when, where, and why for the event to be remembered. You can help by providing context for things you're trying to remember, by imagining people's names and faces in different parts of your house, or at various points along a favorite walk. You'll find it useful to make a mental picture of the thing you are trying to remember, if it lends itself to imagery. In addition to changing the strategies you use to remember something, there are many aids we are all familiar with that can help us remember things more easily. Make lists, organize important things, and plan ahead.

Finally, there's the art of flexible thinking. Challenge your brain! Different people will come up with their own individual solutions. The important thing is to make your brain do some work. Many guides to mental exercises have come on the market. One of the best in this new field of "neurobics" is *Keep Your Brain Alive: 83 Neurobic Exercises* by a noted brain scientist at Duke University, Lawrence Katz, and his colleagues.

Feel Good about Yourself, Keep Control of Your Life

Maintaining these attitudes may be the most important thing you can do. Part of this attitude involves recognizing the stresses in your life, seeking help from others, and maintaining supportive relationships.

Maintain Relationships

Support from family, friends, support groups, and religious affiliations can be your strongest bulwark against disease. In chapter 19, "Stroke: The Brain-Heart Connection," we talked about how depression can predispose people to heart disease and can also complicate the outcome. One study showed that although people who were recovering from heart attacks and had depression had a three- to fourfold risk of dying from their condition, depressed individuals with strong support from their loved ones did not face the same risk.

In studying how connections with other people exert their influence, scientists have zeroed in on the immune system. Their research shows that that among people in chronically stressful situations (such as receiving a diagnosis of cancer or caring for a family member with Alzheimer's disease), the ones who reported higher stress levels and less satisfactory relationships also showed changes in the functioning of several types of white blood cells involved in the immune response. Research is now under way to see how, or if, these changes translate into overall health (and, in the case of cancer, the progress of the disease).

TRY TO PREVENT THE DEVELOPMENT OF DISEASE

An ounce of prevention is worth a pound of cure. No better medical advice ever has been or ever will be given. You can do a lot in your daily life to prevent illnesses that affect the brain.

Perhaps the most prominent area of preventable disease is vascular disease (diseases of the blood vessels of the heart, brain, and other organs). Controlling high blood pressure and high cholesterol, getting rid of excess weight, stopping smoking, and detecting and treating diabetes can have dramatic effects. The number of people in the United States with stroke, for example, is decreasing each year because people are paying attention to those measures. If this trend continues, what had been the killers and disablers of our parents will have much less effect on our children.

An often-neglected step is keeping your alcohol consumption moderate. There is scarcely a disease of the brain that excessive drinking does not make worse. Alcohol is often a response to boredom and isolation, and it can be both a cause and a reaction to depression. Drinking too much increases the chance of falling, impairs memory, interferes with good nutrition, disrupts sleep, and causes weight gain. Alcoholism can mask other diseases, such as depression, Alzheimer's or Parkinson's disease, and make diagnosis more difficult. The best way for someone to avoid problems with alcohol is to be honest about how much he or she is drinking, writing down every drink, for example. This way alcohol can be one of the pleasures of growing older, not a scourge.

If you have not done so already, quit smoking! Fortunately, most people are aware of the hazards of smoking. It contributes to the three most common causes of death in the elderly: cancer, heart disease, and stroke. One of our physician friends once observed, only half jokingly, that if no one smoked, half the physicians in the country would be out of work!

RECOGNIZE DISEASE EARLY

It would be naive to think or to pretend that there are not diseases of the brain in the elderly. But great progress has been made in understanding these disease processes and there are new treatments becoming realities at amazing rates. When a clearly unusual mental or neurological symptom enters the picture, it's important to accept that aging (like any time of life) has disorders that are not like the discomforts or changes that one can handle alone with simple strategies or better exercise or nutrition. More and more it is becoming evident that early recognition of a disease is important. In stroke, for example, knowing the warning signs and getting to the hospital is sometimes the difference between life and death, and often the difference between a good outcome and some degree of disability.

We cannot emphasize enough the positive psychological effect of knowing what's wrong. Uncertainty about one's health is very unsettling. If we clinicians can tell you what's wrong, what can be done about it, and what to expect, these uncertainties can be minimized. Sometimes they can even be eliminated. Serious illnesses like Alzheimer's disease, for example, loom so large in national awareness that the slightest lapse in memory can have us frantic. But as we've discussed, many forms of memory impairment and even dementia are readily treatable.

Signs of illness that should be checked out include the following:

• *Memory problems.* We all have "senior moments" when we cannot come up with the name of a friend or a place. These lapses are normal, and do become more frequent as we get older. However increasing forgetfulness in other areas such as remembering recent events or conversations may not be normal and should be evaluated. Failing memory has many causes, and many are treatable.

• *Changes in attitude and mood.* Depression is a very sneaky process, it creeps up on people. In addition, it is a common misperception that a person will just "snap out of it"—often that doesn't happen. There are particular danger times, such as serious illness or injury, the death of a spouse or close friend, moving to a new location, retiring, changes in financial status, or sometimes just plain loneliness. Look out under these circumstances; you are not made of iron. Get help and use it.

• *Daytime sleepiness.* A change in sleeping pattern, particularly sleepiness during the daytime, often means that something is going on at night that is interfering with sleep—something you may not be aware of. The most common unrecognized problems are sleep apnea and restless legs, both of which are quite treatable.

• *Difficulty getting around.* Difficulties with walking, balancing, getting out of a chair, or writing a letter may spring from numerous causes. They need to be sorted out—Parkinson's disease, essential tremor, or bony disease of the spine can all be diagnosed and treated.

• *Vision and hearing loss.* Changes in hearing and vision are so common in the elderly that it is hard to draw a line between the normal and abnormal. Regardless, if left untreated they can lead to progressive social isolation. The most common causes can be fixed—cataracts by surgery and high-tone deafness with hearing aids. There is no reason for people to put up with a degree of sensory deprivation from these treatable problems.

• *Headaches.* Headaches occurring for the first time, or a changing pattern of headaches, make many people worry that they may have a brain tumor. The chance of such a tumor being present is very small, but the possibility can be immediately ruled out with a simple brain imaging study (a CT scan or an MRI). Why walk around worried when a definitive answer is so easy to obtain?

What's Coming?

We are both members of the Dana Association for Brain Disorders, a group of brain scientists dedicated to the advancement of brain research. This group recently articulated a vision of the future. It's opening statement read as follows:

Imagine a world, the world of 2025—

In which Alzheimer's, Parkinson's, Lou Gehrig's (ALS) diseases, and retinitis pigmentosa and other causes of blindness are commonly detected in their early stages, and are swiftly treated by medications that stop deterioration before significant damage occurs.

In which spinal cord injury doesn't mean a lifetime of paralysis because the nervous system can be programmed to re-wire neural circuits and re-establish muscle movement.

In which drug addiction and alcoholism no longer hold people's lives hostage because easily available treatments can interrupt the changes in neural pathways that cause withdrawal from, and drive the craving for addictive substances.

In which the genetic pathways and environmental triggers that predispose people to mental illness are understood so that accurate diagnostic tests and targeted therapies—including medications, counseling, and preventive interventions—are widely available and fully employed.

In which new knowledge about brain development is used to enhance the benefits of the crucial early learning years and combat diseases associated with aging.

In which people's daily lives are not compromised by attacks of depression or anxiety because better medications are being developed to treat these conditions.

STAY INFORMED

We did not make these statements up; they are optimistic projections based on today's trends in brain research, many of which we have presented in this book. We have also described what changes can be expected as part of normal aging and what are the early indications of disease. You are flooded with other sources of information, some reliable, some not. In the Appendix we have outlined dependable sources about diet, alternative therapies, and diseases. We are sure you can find still other sources of information, but this is a place to start. By protecting your brain as well as using it, you can move through your "second half" with awareness and composure. So mind your brain—it's the only one you've got, so take good care of it.

Appendix

This is not an exhaustive list. We have included books and web sites that we have found to be informative and helpful.

In general, we have chosen web sites that are .org or .gov, and not .com. Many commercial web sites (.com) are often biased toward a specific product or approach to a problem.

We have made specific comments about books, but not web sites. We have chosen web sites that provide information about research and services. Most are also associated with organizations that have local chapters.

GENERAL WEB SITES

These are web sites that act as clearing houses for more specific, disease-oriented web sites.

The Dana Foundation
www.dana.org/brain
745 Fifth Avenue, Suite 700
New York, NY 10151
(212) 223-4040

There are several such sites associated with specific institutes of the National Institutes of Health.

National Eye Institute
www.nei.nih.gov
2020 Vision Place
Bethesda, MD 20892-3655
(301) 496-5248

National Institute on Aging
www.nih.gov/nia/
Building 31, Room 5C27
31 Center Drive, MSC 2292
Bethesda, MD 20892
(301) 496-1752

National Institute on Deafness and
   other Communication Disorders
www.nidcd.nih.gov
31 Center Drive, MSC 2320
Bethesda, MD 20892

National Institute of Mental Health
www.nimh.nih.gov
31 Center Drive, MSC 2320
Bethesda, MD 20892

National Institute of Neurological
   Disorders and Stroke
www.ninds.nih.gov
NIH Neurological Institute
PO Box 5801
Bethesda, MD 20892
(800) 352-9424

There are also web sites associated with organizations that provide general information.

AARP
www.aarp.org
601 E Street, NW
Washington, DC 20049
(800) 424-3410

American Academy of Neurology
www.aan.com
1080 Montreal Avenue
St. Paul, MN 55116
(651) 695-1940

American Psychiatric Association
www.psych.org
1400 K Street NW
Washington, DC 20005
(888) 357-7924
(202) 682-6850 (fax)
apa@psych.org (e-mail)

The U.S. Department of Health and Human Services hosts a site which provides information on diseases and food safety.

www.healthfinder.gov
The U.S. Department of Health and Human Services
200 Independence Avenue, SW
Washington, DC 20201
(877) 696-6775

ALCOHOL

Organizations
National Council on Alcoholism and Drug Dependence (NCADD)
www.ncadd.org
20 Exchange Place, Suite 2902
New York, NY 10005
(212) 269-7797
(800) NCA-CALL
national@ncadd.org (e-mail)

Alcoholics Anonymous
www.aa.org
AA World Services, Inc.
475 Riverside Drive, 11th Floor
New York, NY 10115

ALZHEIMER'S DISEASE

Books

Decoding Darkness: The Search for the Genetic Causes of Alzheimer's Disease by
Rudolph E. Tanzi and Ann B. Parson (Perseus Book Group, October 2000).
An excellent presentation of research relating to the genetics of Alzheimer's
Disease.

*The 36-Hour Day: A Family Guide to Caring for Persons with Alzheimer Disease,
Related Dementing Illnesses, and Memory Loss in Later Life* by Nancy L. Mace and
Peter V. Rabins (Warner Books, Inc., April 2001). A caregiver's guide.
Considered the "Bible" for families giving care to loved ones with Alzheimer's
disease.

Organization

Alzheimer's Association
www.alz.org
919 W. Michigan Avenue, Suite 1100
Chicago, IL 60611-1676
(800) 272-3900
(312) 335-8700
(312) 335-1110 (fax)

AMYOTROPHIC LATERAL SCLEROSIS

Book

Tuesdays with Morrie: An old man, a young man and life's greatest lesson by Mitch
Albom (Doubleday, September 1997). This book has been on the bestseller list
for over three years. An account by a former student of the progressive disease
affecting a beloved teacher.

Organization

The ALS Foundation
www.alsa.org
27001 Agoura Road, Suite 150
Calabasas Hills, CA 91301-5104
(800-782-4747)

BLINDNESS/VISION IMPAIRMENT

Organizations
Research to Prevent Blindness
www.rpbusa.org
645 Madison Avenue, 21st Floor
New York, NY 10022
(800) 621-0026

Lighthouse International
www.lighthouse.org
111 E. 59th Street
New York, NY 10022-1202
(800) 829-0500
(212) 821-9200
(212) 821-9713 (TTY)

BRAIN TUMORS

Organizations
The Brain Tumor Society
www.tbts.org
124 Watertown Street, Suite 3-H
Watertown, MA 02472
(800) 770-8287
(617) 924-9997
(617) 924-9998 (fax)
info@tbts.org (e-mail)

American Brain Tumor Association
www.abta.org
2720 River Road, Suite 146
Des Plaines, IL 60018
(847) 827-9910
(847) 827-9918 (fax)
(800) 886-2282 (patient line)
info@abta.org (e-mail)

CANCER

OncoLink
www.oncolink.com
University of Pennsylvania Cancer Center

Deafness/Hearing Loss

Organizations

Alexander Graham Bell Association for the Deaf and Hard of Hearing
www.agbell.org
3417 Vola Place, NW
Washington, DC 20007-2778
(202) 337-5220
(202) 337-8314 (fax)

Cochlear Implant Association International
www.cici.org
5335 Wisconsin Avenue, NW, Suite 440
Washington, DC 20015-2034
(202) 895-2781
(202) 895-2782 (fax)
info@cici.org (e-mail)

Depression

Book

Understanding Depression by J. Raymond DePaulo with Leslie A. Horvitz (John Wiley & Sons, in press). Sound advice from one of the leaders in the field.

Organizations

Depression and Related Affective Disorders Association (DRADA)
www.med.jhu.edu/drada
Meyer 3-181
600 N. Wolfe Street
Baltimore, MD 21287-7381
(410) 955-4647 Baltimore
(202) 955-5800 Washington, DC
drada@jhmi.edu (e-mail)

National Alliance for Research in Schizophrenia and Depression (NARSAD)
www.narsad.org
60 Cutter Mill Road, Suite 404
Great Neck, NY 11021
(800) 829-8289 (InfoLine)
(516) 829-0091
(516) 487-6930 (fax)
info@narsad.org (e-mail)

National Foundation for Depressive Illness
www.depression.org
PO Box 2257
New York, NY 10116
(800) 239-1265

EXERCISE

Book

Strong Women Stay Young by Miriam E. Nelson and Sarah Wernick (Bantam Books, May 2000). A description of doable exercises and their benefits.

MEMORY

Book

Keep Your Brain Alive: 83 Neurobic Exercises by Lawrence Katz, Manning Rubin, and David Suter (Workman Publishing Company, Inc., April 1999). A challenging book by a first-rate brain scientist.

NUTRITION

Books

The American Pharmaceutical Association Practical Guide to Natural Medicines by Andrea Peirce, John A. Gans, Andrew T. Weil (Introduction) (William Morrow & Co., December 1999). This provides a review of virtually all available natural medicines.

Herbal Medicine: Expanded Commission E Monographs by Mark Blumenthal (Editor), Alicia Goldberg (Integrative Medicine Communication, February 15, 2000). This is a translation of the authoritative German statements about herbal Medicines.

Organization

Nutrition Navigator
www.navigator.tufts.edu

PAIN

Organization

American Chronic Pain Association
www.theacpa.org
PO Box 850
Rocklin, CA 95677
(916) 632-0922
(916) 632-3208 (fax)
ACPA@pacbell.net (e-mail)

PARKINSON'S DISEASE

Book

Parkinson's Disease: A Guide for Patient and Family by Roger C. Duvoisin and Jacob I. Sage (Raven Press, January 1996). A valuable guide for dealing with Parkinson's disease, including a section on exercises to maintain and improve mobility and balance.

Organizations

The National Parkinson Foundation, Inc.
www.parkinson.org
1501 NW Ninth Avenue
Miami, FL 33136-1494
(800) 327-4545
(305) 547-6666
(305) 243-4403 (fax)
mailbox@parkinson.org (e-mail)

The Michael J. Fox Foundation for Parkinson's Research
www.michaeljfox.org

840 Third Street   Grand Central Station
Santa Rosa, CA 95404   PO Box 4777
(800) 708-7644   New York, NY 10163

Parkinson's Disease Foundation
www.pdf.org
710 W. 168th Street, 3rd floor
New York, NY 10032-9982
(800) 457-6676

RESTLESS LEG SYNDROME

Organization

RLS Foundation, Inc.
www.rls.org
819 Second Street, SW
PO Box 7050
Dept WWW
Rochester, MN 55902-2985
(507) 287-6465
(507) 287-6312 (fax)
RLSFoundation@rls.org (e-mail)

Sleep

Book

The Promise of Sleep: A Pioneer in Sleep Medicine Explores the Vital Connection Between Health, Happiness, and a Good Night's Sleep by William C. Dement and Christopher Vaughan (Dell Books, March 2000). A comprehensive book by one of the gurus of sleep research. Very readable and informative.

Organization

National Sleep Foundation
www.sleepfoundation.org
1522 K Street, NW, Suite 500
Washington, DC 20005
(202) 347-3471
(202) 347-3472 (fax)
nsf@sleepfoundation.org (e-mail)

Stroke

Books

The Stroke Recovery Book: A Practical Guide for Patients and Families by Kip Burkman (LPC, May 1998). An excellent presentation of what happens during a stroke and what are the benefits and expectations of rehabilitation.

After Stroke by David M. Hinds and Peter Morris (Thorsons, June 2000). A discussion of the psychological problems of the stroke victim.

Organizations

American Stroke Association (A Division of the American Heart Association)
www.strokeassociation.org
7272 Greenville Avenue
Dallas, TX 75231
(888) 4-STROKE
strokeassociation@heart.org (e-mail)

National Stroke Foundation
www.stroke.org
9707 E. Easter Lane
Engelwood, CO 80112
(800) STROKES
(303) 649-9299
(303) 649-1328 (fax)

Viagra

Book

Viagra: How the Miracle Drug Happened and What It Can Do for You by Robert A. Kloner, Ann M. Holmes, and Jonathan Jarow (M. Evans & Company, Inc., February 1999). A discussion of how Viagra works and what to expect from its use.

Index

acetylcholine, 11, 22
acoustic nerve, tumors and, 201–2
acupuncture for pain, 92
Acyclovir, 101
ADH, 112
age
    acute confusion and, 158, 163–64
    alcohol consumption and, 76–77
    anesthesia and confusion, 160
    balance and, 132–40
    dehydration and confusion, 160
    depression and, 63–65, 73
    dizziness and, 145
    exercise and, 136–37
    falling and, 137–40
    hearing and, 123–27
    language and 128–30
    memory and, 7–10, 13, 22
    migraine and, 94
    pain and, 100–104
    sexual function and, 107–11, 117
    sleep and, 40, 41
    vision and, 120–23
agonist, 215
alcohol consumption, 26, 47, 74–79, 234, 237, 238
    age and, 76–77
    effect on brain, 75–76, 78
    memory loss and, 151
    migraine and, 95
    moderate drinking, 74–75, 78, 274
    positive effects on brain, 236
    sexual function and, 108

    signs of excess, 78–79
    treatments for problems, 77–78
ALD (assisted listening devices), 125, 127
alpha synuclein, 212, 231
ALS (amyoytophic lateral sclerosis), 239, 241–44, 245, 276
Alzheimer, Alois, 166, 169, 171, 179
Alzheimer's disease, 4, 7, 10, 20, 22, 25, 26, 30, 36, 75, 158, 165–87, 192, 194, 274, 275, 276
    behavioral problems in, 173–75, 176
    bladder function and, 116
    caregiver for, 57, 175, 177, 185–87
    depression in, 173–75
    diagnosing, 168–69
    exercise and, 271
    family's role, 175, 177
    first sign of, 167–68
    genetics and, 170–71
    nursing home care, 177, 186
    progression of, 175–77
    research for, 177–79
    resources and options, 185–87, 279–87
    treatment of, 171–73
    vitamin E and, 172–73, 178
Ambien, 50, 160
amino acids, 34
amyloid, 169, 178, 179, 180
amyoytophic lateral sclerosis. See ALS
Amytal, 153–54
aneurysm, 261, 262, 263
angina, 266
angiography, 263

289